D0517232

PRIMAL CUISINE

"Mouthwatering recipes gorgeously photographed, *Primal Cuisine* is an invaluable nutritional health resource you won't want to live without!"

JIMMY MOORE, AUTHOR OF
21 LIFE LESSONS FROM LIVIN' LA VIDA LOW-CARB

"*Primal Cuisine* provides a clear and straightforward guide to any beginner of the primal lifestyle and a fabulous tool for any well-seasoned primal aficionado. Pauli has written a heart-felt yet informative book that I highly recommend."

LAUREN A. NOEL, ND, HOST OF
DR. LO RADIO

"As a passionate advocate for removing gluten from the American diet, Chef Pauli has hit a home run with *Primal Cuisine*."

FRANKIE BOYER, HOST OF
THE *FRANKIE BOYER* SHOW

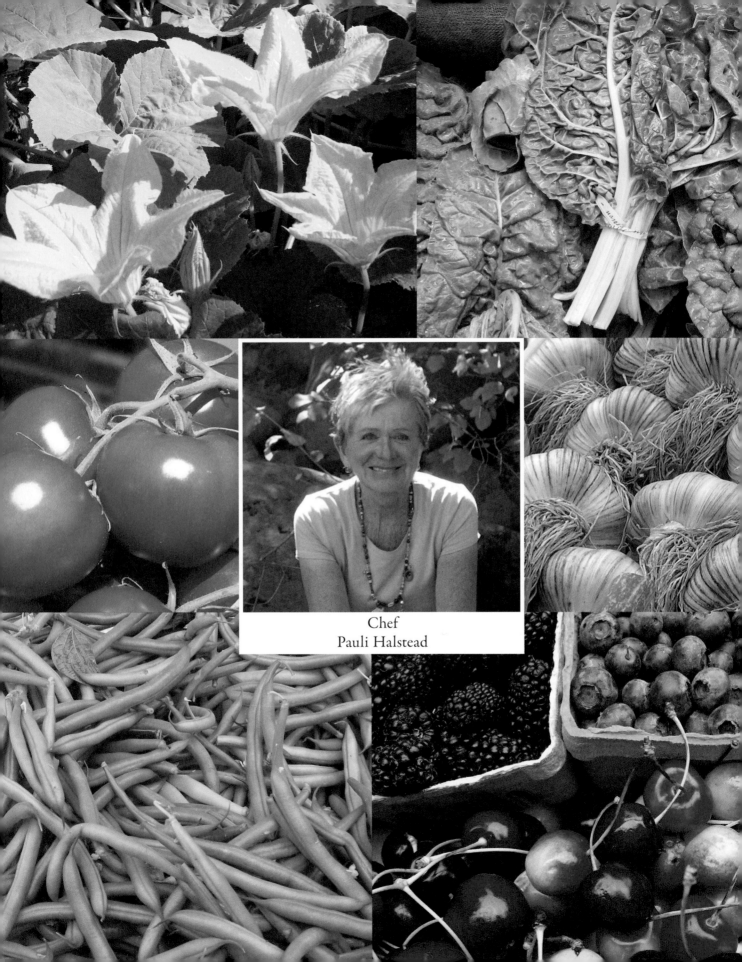

Chef
Pauli Halstead

PRIMAL CUISINE

COOKING
FOR THE
PALEO DIET

PAULI HALSTEAD

Healing Arts Press
Rochester, Vermont • Toronto, Canada

Healing Arts Press
One Park Street
Rochester, Vermont 05767
www.HealingArtsPress.com

Healing Arts Press is a division of Inner Traditions International

Copyright © 2009, 2013 by Pauli Halstead

Originally published in 2009 by Hood River Press under the title *Cuisine for Whole Health: Recipes for a Sustainable Life*

All rights reserved. No part of this book may be reproduced or utilized in any form or by any means, electronic or mechanical, including photocopying, recording, or by any information storage and retrieval system, without permission in writing from the publisher.

Note to the reader: *This book is intended as an informational guide. The remedies, approaches, and techniques described herein are meant to supplement, and not to be a substitute for, professional medical care or treatment. They should not be used to treat a serious ailment without prior consultation with a qualified health care professional.*

Library of Congress Cataloging-in-Publication Data
Halstead, Pauli.
  Primal cuisine : cooking for the paleo diet / Pauli Halstead.
     p. cm.
  Includes index.
  Summary: "Nourishing and innovative paleo recipes to delight your family, impress your guests, and inspire your culinary talents while improving your health." — Provided by publisher.
   ISBN 978-1-59477-486-7 (pbk.) — ISBN 978-1-59477-503-1 (e-book)
  1. Cooking (Natural foods) 2. Health. I. Title.
  TX741.H352 2012
  641.3'02—dc23
                                                                                    2012012924

Printed and bound in the United States by Versa Press, Inc.

10 9 8 7 6 5 4 3 2

Text design and layout by Virginia Scott Bowman
This book was typeset in Garamond Premier Pro, Berkeley Oldstyle, and Gill Sans with Berkeley Oldstyle and Arial used as display typefaces.

To send correspondence to the author of this book, mail a first-class letter to the author c/o Inner Traditions • Bear & Company, One Park Street, Rochester, VT 05767, and we will forward the communication, or contact the author directly at **cuisineforwholehealth@gmail.com**.

◆

In gratitude for my family
Janette and Ray Halstead;
Brothers Bob, Glenn, and Chuck;
Children John, Shannon, and Devon;
Grandson Michael

All things are connected.
Whatever befalls the earth
Befalls the sons of the earth.
Man did not weave the web of life,
He is merely a strand in it.
Whatever he does to the web,
He does to himself.

CHIEF SEATTLE

We actually have the capacity and key information that can allow
us to live longer and healthier than we ever have before in our
long evolutionary history . . . but only if we have the wisdom to
use it.

NORA GEDGAUDAS

CONTENTS

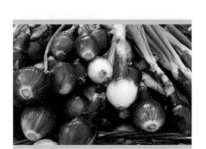

PART 1

THE PRIMAL DIET, A SUSTAINABLE EARTH, AND THE PALEO-FRIENDLY KITCHEN

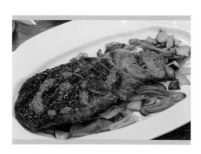

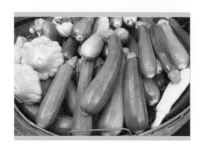

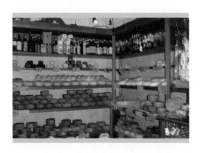

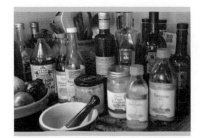

PART 2

RECIPES

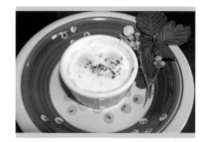

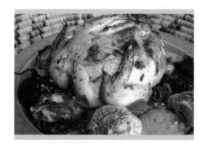

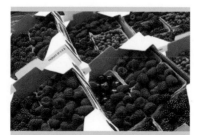

METRIC CONVERSION CHART

For those of you who might use the metric system, I've included
a conversion chart below for your convenience.

WEIGHT		VOLUME		LENGTH	
15 g	½ oz	5 ml	1 teaspoon (tsp)	5 mm	¼ inch
20 g	¾ oz	10 ml	1 dessertspoon (dsp)	1 cm	½ inch
25 g	1 oz	15 ml	1 tablespoon (tbsp.)	2.5cm	1 inch
40 g	1½ oz	20 ml	1 Australian tablespoon	5 cm	2 inch
50 g	2 oz	30 ml	1 fl oz	7.5 cm	3 inch
75 g	3oz	40 ml	1½ fl oz	10 cm	4 inch
100 g	3½ oz	60 ml	2 fl oz	12 cm	5 inch
110 g	4 oz	85 ml	3 fl oz	15 cm	6 inch
125 g	4½ oz	100 ml	3½ fl oz	18 cm	7 inch
150 g	5 oz	125 ml	4 fl oz	20 cm	8 inch
175 g	6 oz	150 ml	5 fl oz	23 cm	9 inch
200 g	7 oz	175 ml	6 fl oz	25 cm	10 inch
225 g	8 oz	200 ml	7 fl oz	28 cm	11 inch
250 g	9 oz	250 ml	8 fl oz	30 cm	12 inch
275 g	10 oz	300 ml	10 fl oz (½ pint)		
300 g	10½ oz	350 ml	12 fl oz		
350 g	12 oz	375 ml	13 fl oz		
400 g	14 oz	400 ml	14 fl oz		
425 g	15 oz	425 ml	15 fl oz (¾ pint)		
450 g	1 lb	450 ml	16 fl oz		
500 g	1 lb 2 oz	500 ml	18 fl oz		
600 g	1¼ lb	600 ml	20 fl oz (1 pint)		
700 g	1½ lb	750 ml	1¼ pints		
750 g	1 lb 10 oz	800 ml	1⅓ pints		
900 g	2 lb	1 liter	1¾ pints		
1 kg	2¼ lb	1.2 liters	2 pints		
1.5 kg	3¼ lb	1.5 liters	2½ pints		
2 kg	4½ lb	2 liters	3½ pints		

OVEN TEMPERATURES

140°C	275°F	Gas 1	Cool
150°C	300°F	Gas 2	Low
160°C	325°F	Gas 3	Moderately low
180°C	350°F	Gas 4	Moderate
190°C	375°F	Gas 5	Moderately hot
200°C	400°F	Gas 6	Hot
220°C	425°F	Gas 7	Hot
230°C	450°F	Gas 8	Very hot

Cooking times used are based on a conventional oven. If you are using a convection oven, set the temperature to 10° to 15°C lower than called for in the recipe.

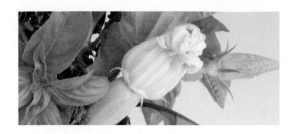

ACKNOWLEDGMENTS

I would like to thank Nora Gedgaudas, author of *Primal Body, Primal Mind: Beyond the Paleo Diet for Total Health and a Longer Life,* who has been extremely generous in allowing me to quote her extensively for this book. With her vast knowledge of how the body functions and the nutritional support it needs, Nora has been able to help me let go of a lifetime of sugar addiction and bad eating habits, which had resulted in hypoglycemia and depression. More important, her kindness and compassion have helped me to achieve optimal health. She is truly a cheerleader and buddy.

Thanks to Dr. Diana Schwarzbein, author of *The Schwarzbein Principle,* and Dr. Mark Hyman, author of *The UltraMind Solution,* and many other authors listed in the recommended reading section at the end of this book, who are helping to bring in to public awareness the importance of diet and its relation to our physical and mental health.

My friend and partner, Curt, was my taste tester and was happy to do it. I asked him to discern the nuances in each of the recipes, and he became quite good at critiquing. Curt was a good subject, as he was used to the normal way some dishes were supposed to taste. I wanted him to see whether the new versions, without the typical sugars or gluten-containing ingredients, tasted as good as the originals. He was amazed at how much better the new versions were and began to prefer desserts that were not overly sweetened.

I would never have written this book if it had not been for my spiritual mentor and friend, Elle Collier Re (Annam), who has been an inspiration and a guiding support since our meeting in Santa Fe in the spring of 2006. I lived with Elle and her significant other, Michael Friend, at HeartGate Sanctuary in Hood River, Oregon, for more than two years, from 2007 to 2009. At HeartGate I began learning the art of forgiveness and unconditional love. This remarkable teacher has helped me let go of the past and learn to live in the "eternal now" presence of love. Elle's teaching is simple: every day is a blessing and an opportunity to love everyone we meet with no exceptions. As far as taking care of the body itself, Elle says we are to help the body and all of its energies to be used for Goodness (good works on Earth). We are to educate ourselves about what our body really needs in the moment. We are to respect our body by taking care of it. And, most important, we are to be grateful.

I would like to acknowledge my family, which includes my three brothers, Bob, Glenn, and Chuck; my three children, John, Shannon, and Devon; and one grandchild, Michael. We have all had our health issues in recent years, and all of the research for this book has been for a purpose: to enable us to understand the past so we can make our *present* as healthy and positive as possible. My goal in writing this book is to create enthusiasm and interest with the recipes so that achieving greater health for ourselves and our families is something that brings joy into daily life.

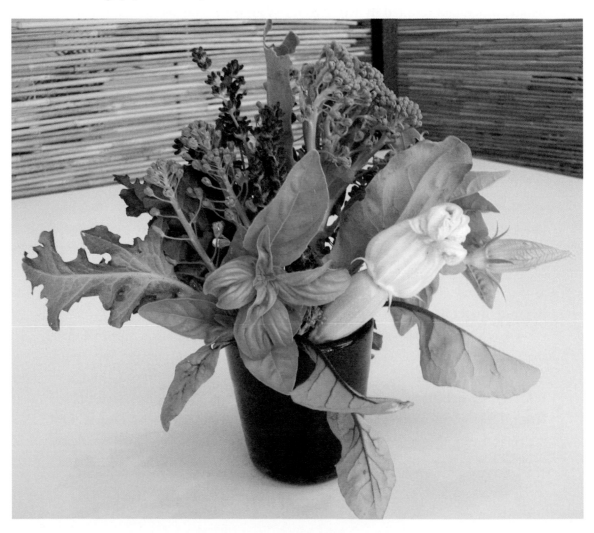

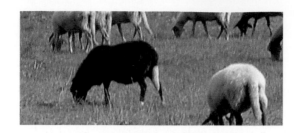

FROM "CAVEMAN COOKING" TO AN EVERYDAY CULINARY "ENCHANTED GROTTO"

By Nora Gedgaudas

At long last, someone wonderful has come along and written the closest thing to a culinary cuisine recipe-guide companion to my own book, *Primal Body, Primal Mind*. With *Primal Cuisine,* chef Pauli Halstead has created a compendium of culinary masterpieces that are sure to please even the most discriminating of primal palates. Having sampled some of Pauli's creations, I have been struck by how memorable they are, even in their relative simplicity. I will never forget her "Thai Salad with Spicy Dressing" made with tender chicken, or "Salmon with Haricots Verts, Eggs, and Nicoise Olives" . . . the stuff that dreams are made of. Mmmmmmm . . . She has turned the principles presented in *Primal Body, Primal Mind* into jaw-dropping, world-class cuisine.

This book itself is a feast for the eyes—gorgeously illustrated—as well as a feast for your palate; it is well designed with practical usage in mind. It can even be used as a daily and weekly meal plan guide. Recipe for recipe, this cookbook is the best I've found so far for promoting both health and sustainability, including sustainability of budget. There is something for everyone in the pages of *Primal Cuisine*. It has been tailored to aid those suffering from gluten sensitivity and other common food-intolerance issues, as well as taking into consideration the growing concerns about GMOs and mercury toxicity.

This book is family friendly, replete with familiar ingredients that most people will have handy in their homes or find easily in their local natural markets. The recipes are easy to follow and are accessible even to those having only the most basic of kitchen skills. At the same time, Pauli chose recipes that would inspire those who enjoy innovative cooking, effectively eliminating boredom in the kitchen and satisfying even the most finicky of taste buds.

Pauli is an experienced gourmet chef, having owned a successful restaurant in San Francisco and an acclaimed catering company in Napa Valley. There is nothing amateurish about her knowledge of food or her creative culinary prowess. These recipes are sufficiently awe-inspiring and elegant to dazzle guests at dinner parties and sufficiently simple to grace your family's everyday table. Pauli is an undisputed master of natural and sustainable healthy cuisine.

Primal foods never tasted so imaginative or inspired. This beautifully written and illustrated book is sure to be a treasured part of your kitchen library for many years to come.

Nora T. Gedgaudas, CNS, CNT, author of *Primal Body, Primal Mind,* is a certified nutritional therapist and neurofeedback specialist with a private practice. A member of the Nutritional Therapy Association, the National Association of Nutritional Professionals, the Nutrition and Metabolism Society, and the Weston A. Price Foundation, she lives in Portland, Oregon.

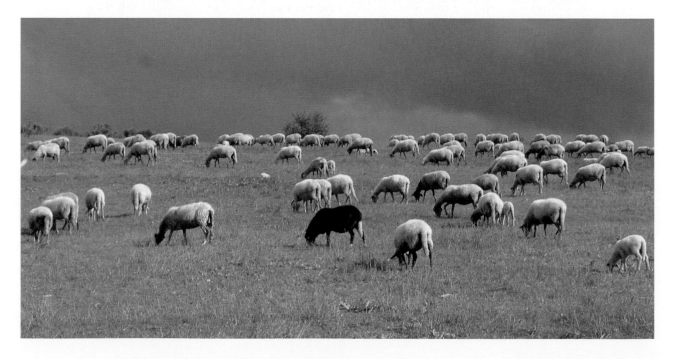

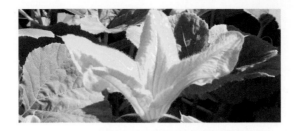

PREFACE

A NOTE TO THE READER

Let food be thy medicine, let medicine be thy food . . .

HIPPOCRATES

Writing this book has been a transformative process. It has made me examine and re-examine all my beliefs about food and what food is for. I have had to let go of all previous ideas of right and wrong eating and what others are doing or not doing with their diets. If anything, the process of deciding where I stood on many issues kept collapsing as I was presented with yet another way to look at things. In this process I have been thoroughly cooked.

I was led to this question: Is it our beliefs about food that make it good or not good for us? The raw food folks (some eat raw meat) believe that their way is the best for optimum health. The vegetarians believe that a plant-based diet is the kindest to the animals with whom we share the planet. But is that really true? We now realize that the commercial cultivation of crops such as grains has eradicated habitat and caused the extinction of many species of animals and birds. The vegans advocate not using any animal products at all or wearing anything made from an animal. Some of the meat-eating people I know are switching to grass-fed meats. Everyone has experts, doctors, and scientists, with published scientific studies, to back up their point of view. So how do we distill all this information to decide what it is we want to feed ourselves?

Some of us who are committed to creating a more sustainable and fair social and global environment are still in a quandary about what to eat, and many of us are still very attached to our food habits. I have noticed everyone has *very* strong opinions about what to eat.

I have come to believe that the true sustenance on which the body thrives is Divine Love, and the reason we overeat is because we feel it is not present. In the process of eating, when it is done consciously, the body fully absorbs the life force that is in the food. We have the innate ability to absorb Divine Love into the very cells and bones in our body if we begin to pay attention. Through our conscious alignment with Divine Love, what we eat gets transmuted, and the result is *energetic love* to be shared and made useful in the world.

When we turn our attention to God in gratitude and love, his love comes pouring back into our bodies, blessing us and sustaining us. Our part is to listen to our body, which requires deep inquiry, to find out what it is asking for in the moment, and this might be different for each person. This is obviously not a "one size fits all" approach; whatever choice a person makes deserves respect. There is no right and wrong, but there is inquiry and dialogue—dialogue with our body and dialogue with others. There will be modifications and changes as we go along. Eating *sustainably* is eating just what our body requires in that precise moment so that the nourishment will carry us and support us in living a life of usefulness. Our gratitude allows us to love God in all things—our food, our planet, ourselves, and each other.

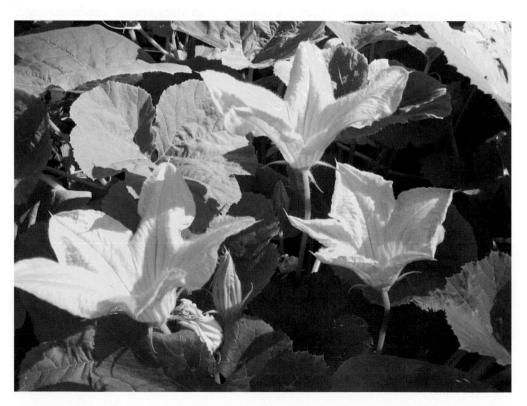

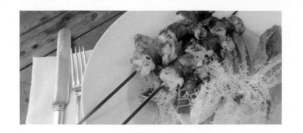

CHOOSING HEALTH, EMBRACING THE PALEO DIET

I'm not going to eat it unless it's delicious. Period! The reason most diets don't work is that they are *boring* and you feel like you're being punished. You can hardly wait until the designated time frame is up and you can return to your old eating habits. Have you ever started a diet and had your energy crash and then become so totally obsessed with food you couldn't think straight? Sounds familiar doesn't it? So what will work? What *will* work is what supports your body energetically in the foods you choose to eat.

Perhaps your body has gone to sleep on you in certain ways. If you are suffering from low energy, a foggy brain, and general malaise, that might be a clue to what doesn't work. You wouldn't put bad motor oil in your car, so why put food in your body that yields a low-energy result or, worse, causes you to get sick? On the other hand, if you begin feeding your body only nutrient-dense foods, these foods have the ability to rebalance, heal, and sustain your precious life.

In 2009, I was right in the middle of writing my first cookbook, *Cuisine for Whole Health,* when a Portland friend of mine handed me yet another book to read and said it would change my approach to what I was writing. I was not pleased, as things were going pretty well, or so I thought. This darned book was *Primal Body, Primal Mind* by Nora Gedgaudas, a Portland-based neurofeedback specialist and board certified nutritional therapist. Nora has extensively studied the Paleolithic diet of our distant ancestors and why it was successful from an evolutionary point of view.

Primal Body, Primal Mind stopped me dead in my tracks. Through it I realized that all humans have the same evolutionary genetics and that our bodies and brains have flourished on certain basic foods for a hundred thousand generations of our evolution. These foods are wild-caught fish and grassfed meats (previously wild meats), organic vegetables, nuts, seeds, and berries. Our bodies and our large human brains evolved on these nutrient-dense foods.

There is strong evidence to support the fact that our distant ancestors did not eat many plants, because they did not cook. Furthermore, only cooking would have removed toxins from the plants and therefore most plants were avoided. We know that intensive cultivation of grains began about 10,000 years ago. Because of this historically recent development we do not *require* grains in our diet, and in fact our bodies have not really adapted genetically to grain consumption. While there has been some discussion, and apparently evidence, that our distant ancestors may have eaten wild grains and plants by pounding them, they did this only as a last resort if no meat was available. Wild meat and fish was the preferred food for sustaining life.

Contemporary humans have been on Earth for about 200,000 years, and during that time we have survived and thrived without the need for processed foods, medical interventions, or pharmaceuticals. At no previous time in history have humans eaten the foods that are now prevalent in the American diet. The American food pyramid is a joke. We are eating food that no longer contains the nutrients necessary for sustaining life and health. Only since the Industrial Revolution has whole food nutrition been replaced by processed "junk" foods, genetically modified plants, and animals supplemented with hormones and antibiotics.

The chemicals, food additives, and genetically modified organisms that have been approved for our food supply by the Federal Food and Drug Administration (FDA) are making us ill. We are now spending billions, possibly trillions, of dollars on health care without addressing the simple fact that many illnesses may be caused by these toxic substances and a nutrient-deficient diet. Scientific facts bear out this theory: the tests have been done and analyzed and the papers have been written and published. The foods we choose to eat (and not eat) have *everything* to do with our health.

Sustainability is one of the buzzwords of our age, but do we include our body as something we consider sustaining? Probably not! We are all hoping we can keep going no matter what we feed ourselves. Our bodies are now screaming at us in a number of different ways: Enough already! In my own experience, after having a lot of bad eating habits over a lifetime, I was suffering from the resulting uncomfortable symptoms, illnesses, depression, low energy, and stress.

I've been a chef and caterer for more than thirty years, beginning with my first restaurant, Pauli's Café, founded in San Francisco in 1975. In 1980 I moved to the Napa Valley and ran a successful catering business, The Best of Everything, until retiring in 2003. In my long culinary career I was cooking what I thought were fabulous and delicious foods. However, my body and brain began deserting me incrementally over the years. My body was letting me know I wasn't taking care of it properly, and I knew I had to make a change.

In 2009 I became a client of Nora's, and after being tested I found out I was hypoglycemic. As a result I decided to reduce the obvious problem-causing carbohydrates and sugars in my diet. Just eliminating refined sugar, honey, and maple syrup was not enough. I also had to eliminate the foods that easily convert to sugar when consumed, like bread, rice, starchy vegetables (potatoes), pasta, and grains. Changing my diet certainly wasn't easy, and it's taken some perseverance, but it's been well worth it. Finally taking responsibility for what I was eating made a huge difference in my health and level of energy. When I began experimenting with recipes based on the Paleo diet, I realized I could have both wonderful cuisine and a healthy body. The two are mutually *inclusive* after all.

We can all live a life that is symptom-free and full of vibrant energy. Many of the diseases affecting Americans today can be cured or greatly alleviated by a change in diet, supplementing with vitamins and minerals, drinking pure filtered water, and detoxifying from heavy metals, yeast overgrowth, and various molds. It has now been scientifically recognized that many diseases, both mental and physical, such as diabetes, obesity, Alzheimer's, chronic fatigue syndrome, ADD/HD, and various depressions, are the result of poor assimilation of food, food allergies, heavy metal toxicity, environmental toxins, and digestive imbalances. Poor diets equal disease and increased medical expenses. It's as simple as that. By making significant dietary changes, our dependence on pharmaceuticals and over-the-counter medications will be greatly reduced and even eliminated. As a result, our medical bills will also decrease.

Simply by changing the way you eat you can improve your health, regain your positive outlook, boost your level of energy, and possibly even live longer. Just imagine what it will be like to live a life where you feel good *all the time*. The purpose of this book is to help you make the necessary changes to a new way of eating, simply and deliciously. By cooking the recipes in this book you will still be eating your favorite foods, but without harmful ingredients, like grains,

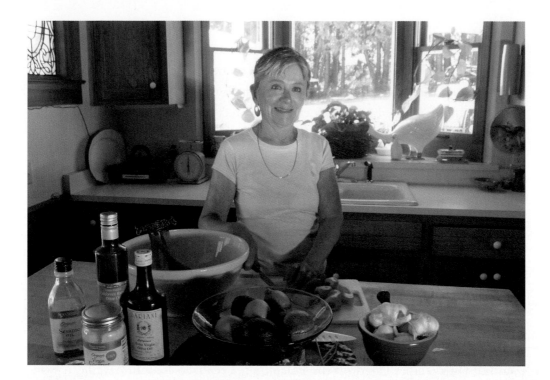

gluten, refined food products, sugar, bad oils and trans-fats, high fructose corn syrup, and preservatives. When you make the recipes they will only taste *better* than before. If you have friends over for dinner they won't notice you've removed harmful ingredients and substituted healthy ones. But they just might be aware they are eating food that is vibrant, delicious, and healthy.

This new cookbook based on the Paleolithic diet offers you facts and information to help you get organized and begin a path to optimum health. In addition to the background information and recipes, I have also included a Resources section at the end of the book, which is rich with healthy sources of the basic foods that compose primal cuisine, information sources for further research, and recommended reading materials. Please keep your mind open and test everything by how you are feeling once you are eating according to the Paleo diet. In choosing toxin-free foods you will be making choices that are also supportive of a healthy planet Earth and a better future for our children and the generations to come. We certainly want to leave the Earth in a better condition than we found it.

There's work to do and each of us—by eating the evolutionarily successful primal diet—will make a positive contribution. This book will help make doing so an interesting, fun, and rewarding adventure.

PART 1

...

THE PRIMAL DIET, A SUSTAINABLE EARTH, AND THE PALEO-FRIENDLY KITCHEN

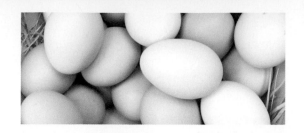

THE PALEO DIET

GOOD NUTRITION IS A WAY OF LIFE

In 1952, when I was six years old, our family moved from Minnesota to the San Joaquin Valley of California. The 1950s were the time when food "inventions" became popular and were being consumed by an unaware American public as safe (approved by the FDA). My early diet, and the diet of my three younger brothers, consisted of these *manufactured food products:* Velveeta Cheese, Crisco, margarine, and Skippy peanut butter (hydrogenated vegetable oils); bottled salad dressings with artificial flavors and preservatives; and white bread and breakfast cereals containing mostly refined grains and *lots* of sugar. We grew up eating commercially raised meat and poultry, which were fed grains grown with chemical fertilizers and pesticides.

These "new" foods were a far cry from the natural and nourishing foods my mother was raised on in the small town of Sartell, Minnesota. Her father, Charles Sartell, had one of the biggest gardens in town during the Depression, and he shared the extra vegetables with his neighbors. Mother's family had rich sources of wholesome dairy products, and they had access to barnyard chickens and eggs. During the Depression, when meat sources were scarce, they ate hunted meat (some squirrel I hear). For fish they just walked across the street to the Mississippi River. Even during the Depression, when my grandfather lost his lumber mill, their diet remained relatively high in essential nutrients.

After we moved to California and began eating the new food inventions, my mother became ill with schizophrenia, which she had for the remainder of her life. It became my lifelong quest to discover what caused my mother's illness. During the course of this inquiry, I came across three books that discussed possible triggers for my mother's illness; these books also influenced the way this cookbook came about and why the recipes contain specific ingredients while leaving out others.

The first book is *The Schwarzbein Principle,* written by Dr. Diana Schwarzbein, a respected authority on the treatment of diabetes, addictions, weight loss, and the prevention and reversal of the degenerative diseases of aging. She also subspecializes in metabolism, diabetes, osteoporosis, menopause, and thyroid conditions. According to Dr. Schwarzbein, type 2 diabetes can be greatly alleviated and even cured by proper diet.

The second book—*The UltraMind Solution* by Dr. Mark Hyman—caught my attention in 2009 when I lived in Hood River, Oregon. After reading his book I began to suspect that my mother's schizophrenia was the result of possible food allergies, a poor diet lacking in essential nutrients, and smoking (which she started as a teenager). Dr. Hyman's book reveals the epidemic of brain problems (broken brains) we are facing as a society today. These brain problems include ADD/HD, autism, and Asperger's syndrome, bipolar disorder, anxiety, insomnia, mood swings, Alzheimer's, Parkinson's, and schizophrenia. According to Dr. Hyman these illnesses are not the result of problems originating *inside* our brains, and we are not suffering from a Prozac deficiency. Rather, these conditions result from continually ingesting toxic foods and breathing in and absorbing environmental pollutants. These food toxins and pollutants then cross the blood-brain barrier, which is much more permeable than originally thought. The many industrial toxins released into the biosphere affect all of us in many ways, especially our delicate brains. To make matters worse we are being prescribed "invented pharmaceuticals" to treat mental illness, but these "cures" come with even more detrimental side effects.

Also in 2009 I discovered the third important book in my journey—*Primal Body, Primal Mind* by Nora Gedgaudas. It was in this book that I learned that a genetic disorder known as pyroluria, which runs in our family, may have also contributed to the onset of mother's schizophrenia. Pyroluria causes a profound vitamin B_6 and zinc deficiency. Vitamin B_6 and zinc are essential for proper brain function. It has now been scientifically proved that brain allergies and the lack of certain nutrients will contribute to the onset of many mental illnesses, including schizophrenia. High concentrations of mercury in the body also block the absorption of zinc. Due to the continued burning of coal as a source of planetary energy, we are all now exposed to high levels of mercury in the atmosphere. Indeed, mercury is now showing up even in breast milk. Evidence from scientific research and statistics (not to mention our national health costs) indicates that most of our population is suffering from a variety of physical and mental problems due to poor nutrition and toxins in our food. For my mother, the combination of a genetic condition, a low-nutrient diet, smoking, and possible environmental toxins created a perfect storm that resulted in the onset of schizophrenia, because any one of these could be a trigger for mental illness.

All of the authors who influenced this cookbook—Dr. Diana Schwarzbein, Dr. Mark Hyman, Nora Gedgaudas, and others—advocate eating a diet free from chemical food additives, refined grain products, sugars, and trans-fats, in other words, *free from prepackaged food products*. Dr. Hyman and Ms. Gedgaudas are also strong proponents of eating animals and dairy products that are exclusively *grassfed* or *pastured,* which means raised out of doors. The meat, fats, and dairy products of animals that are entirely grassfed are of utmost importance to our diet because they retain essential nutrients, most importantly the omega-3 fatty acids and l-tryptophan, an essential amino acid that makes serotonin in the body. Our current American diet is sorely lacking in these essential nutrients, and we now have to pay extra attention to make sure we include meat, fish, and dairy foods that contain all of the essential nutrients in our diet. According to Gedgaudas, "Few are aware that omega-3 fatty acids, which include alpha-linolenic acid, EPA and DHA, are easily the single most deficient nutrient in the modern Western diet. Insufficient intake of this vital and essential dietary component is linked with virtually every modern disease process, weight problem, affective disorder, and learning disability"(page 96).

Fortunately, having optimum nutrition to fuel your life is actually easier than you think. The best way to begin is to make the decision that you are truly committed to your health and then start taking the steps based on that decision. Good nutrition is a *way* of life. Once you are on this way and begin to experience the lasting health benefits of eating nutrient-dense protein, healthy fats, and organic whole vegetables, you will never again go back to your former eating habits.

THE PALEO DIET IS GOOD FOR THE EARTH

In feeding our bodies according to the Paleo diet, we are also taking care of our planet Earth as well. For instance, by eliminating grains and grain-fed meat from our diet, we are conserving precious water. It takes huge amounts of water to grow grains. The mostly genetically modified grains (GMOs) that are used for feed are raised with additional petrochemicals and fertilizers, which ruin our soil and create disaster in the environment. Commercially raised animals are kept in unsanitary conditions on vast feedlots. These animals live under deplorable conditions, which we, in good conscience, cannot support. During what is known as their "finishing time" (when they are fed grains) they are prone to illness, so they are given hormones and antibiotics. Our rivers and oceans are now filled with these runoff antibiotics and chemicals.

Every food choice we make now either contributes to our global environmental problems or helps to eradicate them. We must choose, and *time is of the essence*. We can no longer afford to be oblivious to the maintenance of a healthy biosphere. Specifically, it is important to:

• purchase meats that are entirely grassfed (no grain finishing at all) and request that your grocery store carry these meats;
• choose organic free-range or *pastured* chickens and turkeys when you can find them, and, once again, let your grocer know that you want to have these items in the store;
• purchase line-caught wild fish that are not on the endangered species list as your contribution to saving the oceans for future generations; and
• buy organic foods—organic foods, by law, are not genetically modified.

Sources of these foods are listed in the Resources section at the end of the book. It may seem like a big sacrifice to make significant dietary changes, but the benefits for the *entire Earth* go beyond what you can imagine. We must begin to take into account the global impact of all of our purchases, especially food, that we have to buy every day. One of the main reasons to buy organic foods is that the toxic petrochemicals used to grow crops cause illnesses for many farm workers and their children around the world every year. These biohazards also ruin our soil. It takes years to rebuild soil that has been damaged by petrofertilizers. If you ever fly over California you will see huge areas that have become ugly, dead wastelands due to the use of these chemicals.

The Sacramento River Delta, which is the Western Hemisphere's largest river delta and the stopping place of many bird species, is now in severe decline due to pollutants and the diversion of water from the Sacramento River to southern California. To lose the delta would be a major environmental catastrophe. The effect these poisons have on migrating birds and wildlife has led to the extinction of thousands of species, and they just may be slowly eradicating us as well.*

---

*See "The Delta Crisis," http://water4fish.org/delta-crisis.

It's apparent that only we as individuals can improve our health by what we choose to eat. We can no longer depend on doctors, our government, or our over-burdened health care system to help us. We can no longer ignore the facts being brought so clearly to our attention. Our very lives, and possibly our continued evolution, depend on our choices.

THE PRIMAL HUMAN DIET, OUR EVOLUTIONARY HERITAGE

By analyzing ancient human remains and studying the diets of modern-day hunter-gatherers, evolutionary biologists have gained insights into the ancestral human diet. All ancestral diets shared certain key foods, which were limited to wild animals (especially the brains, bone marrow, fats, and organs), fish and shell-fish, foraged wild plants, eggs, insects, nuts, seeds, and wild berries. The primitive diet provided the nutrient-dense balance for the critical metabolic processes that allowed our ancestors to thrive, reproduce, and pass on their genes to subsequent generations. According to many studies there is now much supporting evidence that the diet of our distant ancestors can provide a guide to the proper nutrition for modern humans. After all, the primitive diet was what our bodies and large brains flourished on; it was the basis for our evolutionary success.

Our species are hunter-gatherers. Certain indigenous groups that were studied during the twentieth century had very similar hunter-gatherer diets, at least prior to their adoption of the Western diet of refined, processed foods. One of the most famous studies of indigenous nutrition was done by Weston A. Price, D.D.S., author of *Nutrition and Physical Degeneration*. During the 1920s and '30s Dr. Price and his wife, Florence, traveled the world, studying isolated groups such as Irish fishermen, Swiss villagers, tribal Africans, Eskimos, Pacific Islanders, Australian Aborigines, and North and South American Indians. He compared the groups who followed their traditional diets—which provided them with good health, sound bodies, and perfect teeth and bones—to those groups who had already been influenced by the consumption of the Western diet. In every instance the groups who had adopted the Western diet soon developed misshapen bones, rampant tooth decay, and mal-formed dental arches (which resulted in crooked teeth), as well as a host of other illnesses, including tuberculosis. Their children also showed these signs of malnutri-tion from the very beginning of their lives, and it soon became evident that genetic deterioration took place after the adoption of the Western diet.

From his extensive research covering six continents, Dr. Price concluded that a diet composed of whole, mineral-rich foods, including sufficient fat-soluble activators found exclusively in animal fats, can provide continuing generations of parents and children with perfect teeth and bone structure and freedom from degenerative diseases and mental illness.

Our hunter-gatherer ancestors ate wild meat and fish and their accompanying fats (high in omega-3 fatty acids) and small amounts of foraged plants, seeds, and nuts. In fact 35 to 50 percent of their dietary intake was made up of the nutrient-rich fats, which retained all the necessary vitamins and minerals, and which provided nourishment to the cells in the body. It has now been scientifically proved that we need these "good" fats and dietary cholesterol to make our bodies and brains function at optimum levels of health.

Today we have accepted that whole grains are the "superfood," and they have formed the base of the American food pyramid. But are they really that healthy? We use these grains to fatten our farm animals, and it is obvious they are making us fat as well. They are now known to be a contributing factor to our mineral-deficient diet. Grains leach minerals from soil and also our bones. There is now much evidence to support the theory that the consumption of grains has caused nutritional stress and has negatively impacted human health.

Historically, the first major change in the human diet began with the cultivation of grains. Pulitzer Prize–winner Jared Diamond, author of *Collapse,* has called the cultivation of grains "the worst mistake in the history of the human race." Cultivation of grains and the advent of animal husbandry led to a widespread replacement of the traditional hunter-gatherer diet with cereal grains and dairy.

Subsequently, the Industrial Revolution led to the onset of advances in crop manipulation, intensive animal-rearing practices, and food processing, all of which radically reduced both the qualitative and quantitative balance of omega-3 fatty acids in the food supply. All these drastic changes in the human diet have occurred in less than two hundred years, which is an insufficient time for genetic adaptation to take place. As a result, people eating the Western diet are no longer consuming omega-3 essential fatty acids and other nutrients within genetically optimal ranges.

We know that all the essential nutrients are important for maintaining critical metabolic processes. These nutrient deficits are playing a major role in the deteriorating health of the American public. Two books—*Pottenger's Cats* by Francis M. Pottenger, M.D., and *Nutrition and Physical Degeneration* by Weston

A. Price, D.D.S.—make it abundantly clear that an optimally healthy life is greatly compromised by a diet devoid of essential nutrients.

What does all this mean for us? Well, we can eliminate grain consumption from our diet and see if some of our illnesses decrease. Grains, when consumed, easily convert to sugar (glucose) that, when not immediately utilized, is then stored in the body as fat. The American epidemic of diabetes, obesity, gluten intolerance, Celiac disease, Alzheimer's, autism, ADD/HD, and major depressions, as well as many other illnesses, is now being linked to our consumption of grains. We must recognize this fact and wean ourselves from all processed foods, which are mostly grain-based. We can return to the successful evolutionary diet of our ancestors by eating exclusively grassfed meat, sustainably fished "wild" seafood, pastured dairy and poultry products, organic produce, nuts, seeds, and berries.

THE BIG *FAT* LIE

The Lipid Hypothesis is the medically and scientifically *unsubstantiated* theory that ingested fat causes heart disease. This theory has been cast in stone by the American Medical Association, and we've been indoctrinated that cholesterol is the worst evil of our modern times. To lower cholesterol, physicians, following the advice of the pharmaceutical companies, have prescribed Lipitor and other statin drugs, which have many side effects. But there are now decades of epidemiological studies that show *no correlation* between saturated fat consumption, high cholesterol levels, and heart disease. France, for example, has one of the highest levels of dietary fat consumption in the form of butter, cheese, and animal fats, but the French have significantly lower coronary heart disease than we Americans.

The famous Framingham Heart study, which began in 1948, attempted to examine the Lipid Hypothesis. It revealed that *declining* cholesterol levels in people over fifty were associated with *increases* in overall mortality and death from cardiovascular disease. Yet people who are proponents of the Lipid Hypothesis still refer to this study in an attempt to prove the link between high cholesterol and coronary heart disease. In fact, Dr. William Castelli, the director of the Framingham study, found that the *more* saturated fat a person ate, the lower their serum cholesterol became. Furthermore, he found that those who ate the most cholesterol, saturated fat, and calories actually weighed the least. They were also the most physically active.

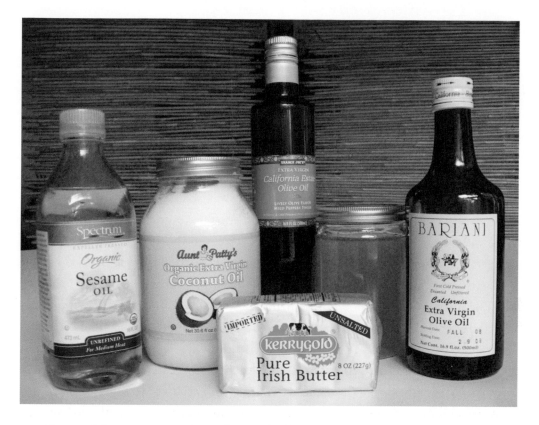

George Mann, a researcher who studied the Masai people of Africa, declared the Lipid Hypothesis possibly the biggest health diversion of this century and perhaps the greatest scam in the history of medicine. The Masai are known to be one of the healthiest peoples on Earth. Their diet is exclusively meat, milk, and cow's blood. Their cholesterol levels are some of the lowest known, and they have no heart disease.

Studies of other modern indigenous tribes, who were still consuming their original diets, yielded similar findings despite consumption of sometimes up to 400 grams of animal fat per day. These people, unlike most Americans, have no rheumatoid arthritis, heart disease, cancer, chronic and degenerative diseases, or high blood pressure. Coconut oil, which is more highly saturated than butter and other animal fats, is the staple food of many Pacific Island groups. Cardiovascular disease and other degenerative diseases are absent in these populations even though 35 to 50 percent of their diet consists of coconut oil. The Okinawan Japanese people are the *longest living people on Earth*. Of those Japanese groups studied, those who ate the most eggs, dairy products, and fish had a 28 percent lower risk of stroke than those who ate the least.

How did we arrive at this big fat misunderstanding? By experimenting on rabbits, of course. When researchers fed fat to rabbits, animals that eat vegetables and not fat, they died. Subsequently, when the fat-feeding experiments were done on carnivores like cats and dogs, no damage resulted. Historically humans are carnivores, not vegetarians (sorry vegetarians and vegans). Simply put, high amounts of animal protein and cholesterol are readily metabolized by carnivorous animals (humans).

As carnivores, our ancestors had to walk and hunt for food, so it was either feast or famine much of the time. Also, food was shared communally with the tribe, and many times there probably wasn't enough to go around. Since starvation was a constant companion, fat was necessary for survival and to stave off hunger. Fat is satiating, and our ancestors consumed the fattiest portions of animals first, such as the brains, bone marrow, and organ meats.

The human body *required* protein and fats to evolve. *Only animal fats* provide the cholesterol the human body and brain require. Cholesterol is a life-sustaining substance, and we need it for our physical and mental health. In *Primal Body, Primal Mind,* Nora Gedgaudas asserts the value of cholesterol.

> Cholesterol is a vital substance in the human body. Using cholesterol, the body produces a series of stress-combatting hormones and mediates the health and efficiency of the cell membranes. . . . Cholesterol is also essential for brain function and development. It forms membranes inside cells and keeps cell membranes permeable. It keeps moods level by stabilizing neurotransmitters and helps maintain a healthy immune system. No steroidal hormone can be manufactured without it, including estrogen, progesterone, testosterone, adrenaline, cortisol, and dehydroepeiandrosterone (DHEA). (pages 76–77)

Every cell in our body needs cholesterol, and, more importantly, life is not possible without it. In fact low blood cholesterol can be fatal. The National Heart, Lung, and Blood Institute held a conference to explore researchers' findings on this very subject. There was much evidence to link low blood cholesterol levels with the rise in various cancers, hemorrhagic stroke, and respiratory and digestive diseases. In light of these findings, Nora points out:

> *Despite the body's ability to manufacture its own cholesterol it is very critical to supplement cholesterol in the diet.* Historically the human diet has always

contained significant amounts of cholesterol. Restricting or eliminating its intake indicates a crisis or famine to the body. The result is the production of a liver enzyme called *HMG-CoA reductase,* which, in effect, then overproduces cholesterol from carbohydrates in the diet. Consuming carbohydrates in the diet, while decreasing cholesterol intake, guarantees a steady overproduction of cholesterol in the body. The only way to switch this overproduction off is to consume an adequate amount of dietary cholesterol and back off the carbs. (page 77)

Instead of avoiding all fats, we need to be choosing the good fats. What is considered a good fat? A "good" fat is a traditional fat like butter (from exclusively grassfed cows), animal fats (also from exclusively grassfed animals), and cold-pressed traditional oils like coconut, sesame, palm, olive, avocado, and flax. Good oils contain essential fatty acids (omega-3 and -6) and are necessary in the diet to maintain optimum health. Fatty acids are strong antioxidants, which help boost the immune system and actually help the body burn excess fat.

Using good fats in our diet is necessary for weight loss. When you eat a combination of good fats throughout the day, and in sufficient quantities, your cravings for carbohydrates will diminish and your blood sugar will remain stable. Eating sensibly will become the norm. It is essential to know that cooked oils cannot be broken down easily by the body. As a result, they promote weight gain and may lead to many health problems. The best way to avoid cooked oils is to not eat foods that are fried in commercial vegetable oils.*

An important thing to remember here is that fats from *exclusively* grassfed and pastured animals, which include the fats in the meat, butter, cheese, whole milk, cream, and eggs replicate the diet of our ancestors in delivering protein, vitamins, minerals, omega-3 fatty acids, and essential amino acids to the cells of our bodies. When commercially raised animals are fed grains, the omega-3 fatty acids are converted to omega-6 fatty acids, and the balance of omega-3s in our diet is lost as a result.

---

*An important article to read is "The Oiling of America" by Sally Fallon, M.A., author of *Nourishing Traditions: The Cookbook that Challenges Politically Correct Nutrition and the Diet Dictocrats.* The article gives a detailed description of which fats and oils are good for us and why. She also documents the politics behind the cholesterol theory of heart disease as advanced by the commercial vegetable-oil industry.

FOOD FOR THOUGHT:
DAILY PROTEIN REQUIREMENTS

So, how much protein does the body need? There are a couple of things to keep in mind. First, adequate dietary fat is required by the body in order to metabolize protein, so you need to eat sufficient fat and protein *together*. Second, a diet *excessively high* in lean protein can be toxic. It is not very well known that if protein is eaten to excess, then the excess will convert to sugar (glucose), which is then converted to fat. So no more big steaks please!

With these two guidelines in mind, we can turn to Nora for specifics: "For most adults the RDA, roughly 0.8 g per kilogram (2.2 pounds) of *ideal* body weight (e.g., 150-pound ideal body weight (68 kg) × .8 g = 54 g), is probably sufficient for 97.5 percent of the adult population (one of the rare RDAs worth paying some attention to)" (page 195). This translates to somewhere between 45 and 60 grams of actual protein per day for most adults. For athletes needing to retain lean tissue mass and peak physical performance, the figure is closer to roughly 60 and 80 grams of protein per day. Also, please note that pregnant women and growing children—both need sufficient protein to grow properly—should not restrict their protein or fat intake. If you have any question about how much protein you should be getting, it's best to consult with a qualified medical practitioner before significantly changing your diet.

Protein is best utilized by the body when consumed in divided amounts during the day, not exceeding 25 grams at a given meal. The recipes in this book are adjusted to keep the protein at each meal within the 25 gram limit, but its best to figure out how much you are consuming at each meal to make sure you do not exceed the recommended daily limits. With the table below you will be able to determine the quantity of protein you will want to have at each meal, including protein from complete (animal) and plant sources. When it comes to protein content in vegetables and legumes, it is important to keep in mind that though you might be getting protein from these incomplete (nonanimal) sources, there are drawbacks to relying on these types of foods entirely for your protein intake. According to Nora, "quality protein is found exclusively in animal-source foods. Combining vegetarian protein sources, such as beans and brown rice, for instance, to create complete protein still makes for a dominantly starchy food, yielding far more starch than protein, despite the combined, more complete amino acid profile, and in no way does this imply protein sufficiency." By using the tables below, you should be able to track how many starchy versus nonstarchy vegetables you should be eating in addition to your meat intake. Including vegetables is still important—eating the vegetables with the protein and the good fats will make you feel satiated longer. Eating less of these precious and *expensive* protein sources is also going to be a huge savings. Still, you will not be suffering from insufficient protein in your diet. By eating the Paleo diet you will be maximizing your nutrient intake while finding that your food dollar stretches further. And that's a very good thing.

The following tables are adapted, with the author's permission, from *Primal Body, Primal Mind* (pages 314 and 315). There, Nora notes that "the source for the information . . . is the USDA Nutrient Database for Standard Reference," and "for the following sources of complete protein, please note that the amount of protein varies with fat content. More fat equals less protein per serving. The following numbers are approximations."

PROTEIN CONTENT BASED ON A 3-OUNCE SERVING

- Egg (medium): 6 g
- Cheese (cheddar): 25 g
- Roast chicken: 25 g
- Sausage: 12 g
- Beef burger: 20 g
- Liver: 23 g
- Turkey: 25 g
- Tuna: 22 g
- Ground beef (lean): 24 g
- Chicken breast: 25 g
- Salmon: 22 g
- Duck (roasted): 24 g
- Fish: 21 g
- Roast beef: 28 g
- Other meats (average): 25 g
- Ham: 18 g
- Corned beef: 26 g
- Sirloin steak: 24 g
- Shrimp: 18–21 g
- Ground beef (regular): 23 g
- Spareribs (lean): 22 g
- Lobster: 17 g
- Feta cheese: 12 g
- Whole-milk yogurt (8 oz): 7 g

PROTEIN CONTENT IN INCOMPLETE OR PLANT SOURCES OF FOODS

- Walnuts (¼ cup): 5 g
- Cashews (¼ cup): 5 g
- Brazil nuts (¼ cup): 5 g
- Peanuts (¼ cup): 9.5 g

- Peanut butter (2 tbs): 8 g
- Pine nuts (¼ cup): 7.5 g
- Oatmeal (1 cup): 6 g
- Pinto beans (¼ cup): 3.5 g
- Tabouli (3 oz): 3 g
- Lentils (½ cup): 9 g
- Brown rice (½ cup): 2.5 g
- Broccoli (½ cup): 2.5–3 g
- Coconut milk (1 cup): 6 g
- Almonds (¼ cup): 7.5 g
- Sunflower seeds (¼ cup): 6.5 g
- Black beans (¼ cup): 4.5 g
- Chickpeas (¼ cup): 4 g
- Quinoa (½ cup): 4.5 g
- Tempeh (½ cup): 20 g
- Stir-fried vegetables (½ cup): 2 g
- Spinach (½ cup): 2.5 g

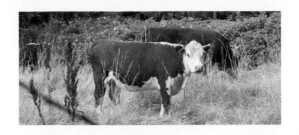

SUSTAINABLE BODY, SUSTAINABLE EARTH

Few human endeavors have as much impact on our planet as the cultivation of food. When you go to the grocery store and see one stack of red tomatoes next to another stack of red tomatoes labeled "organic," and before you choose the cheaper tomatoes, take a moment to consider how they are grown. Conventional tomatoes begin life in a greenhouse, usually in a *synthetic starter* fertilizer. When the plants are large enough the tomatoes are moved to a field that has been treated with approximately 400 to 600 pounds per acre of additional chemical fertilizers. Many tomato plants are also sprayed with fungicides, which are highly toxic to fish and birds.

These chemicals wind up in our groundwater, rivers, and deltas. They wind up in our food, bodies, and breast milk. Almost half a million farmworkers are poisoned by exposure to pesticides every year.

In contrast, the organic method of tomato growing goes something like this: In the fall the land usually gets some kind of cover crop to provide nutrients and organic matter to the soil. The young tomato plants are started in a greenhouse using a mixture of compost, peat moss, fish emulsion, and seaweed extract (sounds good enough to eat). Composted chicken manure, limestone, and potash are used instead of a chemical fertilizer. After planting the tomatoes in the ground, the beds are then covered with straw mulch to keep down the weeds.

When you buy organic produce you are buying a whole farming system that is more labor intensive and not harmful to the environment. Wouldn't you pay a little more for that peace of mind and contribution to our precious planet? Remember that the cost of buying organic foods may be more, but you will no longer be buying *expensive*—and environmentally unsustainable— prepackaged foods, beverages, pastries, ice cream, and bottled salad dressings.

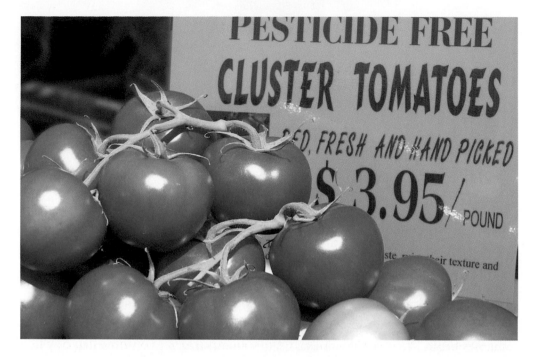

And this "expense" is not just monetary, it is costing our planet. It is essential at this time in our history that we do not continue to compromise our food sources and our water, soils, and air. We must completely change our agricultural practices to preserve our soils, conserve our precious water supply, and remove toxins from our oceans and biosphere.

SOIL DEPLETION IS NUTRIENT DEPLETION

One of the most serious problems confronting us now is the depletion of minerals from our soils. This threat ranks right up there with global warming as an issue that needs our immediate attention and a strong plan for change. Cutting down trees for agriculture and failure to replenish soils has led to the collapse of civilizations. At present the United States has lost approximately 50 million acres of topsoil with another 100 million acres at risk. This is due to poor farming practices and the cultivation of monocrops such as corn, wheat, and soy, all of which deplete nutrients from the soil.

There is now much data on the subject of soil depletion and subsequent animal deterioration. When livestock are fed a diet of grains grown from nutrient-deficient soils, it stands to reason this diet will not provide adequate nourishment for the animals. Subsequently, if we are eating these animals and their milk, cheese, butter, and egg products, then consequently these foods will not contain the essential minerals and nutrients to promote our health, either. Therefore, we *must* feed our farm animals grasses that are grown in nutrient-rich soils. These grasses are high in omega-3 fatty acids and are also rich sources of minerals as well as vitamins E, A, and beta carotene. Eating animals or their products that have been raised *exclusively* on grass will significantly improve our health.

DEFINING *GRASSFED* AND *PASTURED*

The term *grassfed* is applied to ruminants—which include cattle, bison, yak, goats, and sheep—that have consumed nothing but mother's milk and fresh grass or dried grass hay for the duration of their lives, from birth to slaughter. For grassfed nonruminants such as pigs and poultry, grass is still a significant part of their diets. *Pastured* refers to animals, including ruminants and poultry, that are raised out of doors, on a natural diet that includes some grass but also bugs, seeds, and additional organic feed. Almost any food animal we consume can be raised partially or entirely on grass.

There are many health benefits of eating exclusively grassfed and pastured animal products. First of all they are leaner (lower in fats), and the fats they do

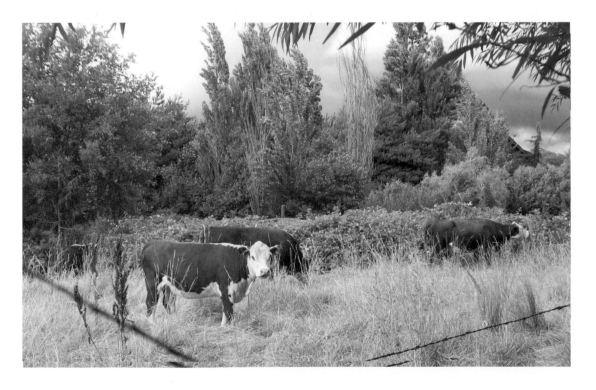

GRASS FED BEEF

Always Naturally Raised With

- No Antibiotics
- No Added Hormones
- No Animal By Products

IT'S WHAT'S FOR DINNER.°

PASTURE RAISED LAMB

Always Naturally Raised With

- No Sub-therapeutic Antibiotics
- No Added Hormones
- No Animal By Products

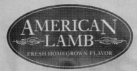

contain are much healthier than fats from commercially raised grain-fed animals. The reason for this is that fats retain toxins, and when the commercially raised animals are fed antibiotics, hormones, and pesticide-laden grains these substances stay in the fat and are then consumed by an unaware public. When farm animals are raised on lush green grass, they absorb vital nutrients, vitamins, and minerals into their flesh, fat, and bones. Grassfed meat and the accompanying fats are richer in antioxidants, including vitamins C and E, and beta carotene. Also, they do not contain added hormones, antibiotics, or other drugs. In addition, the risk of infection by *E. coli* in these products is virtually eliminated because pastured animals *walk away* from their excrement. I'm sure you've seen cows in commercial feed lots standing around in their own waste. *That* is the *E. coli* problem.

Meat from grassfed animals has anywhere from two to four times more omega-3 fatty acids than from grain-fed animals. As mentioned above, omega-3 fatty acids play a vital role in the functioning of every cell in the body; they are essential for a healthy heart and a superbly functioning brain. Omega-3s are significant in *lowering* cholesterol and blood pressure. People with a high intake of omega-3s in their diet are 50 percent less likely to suffer heart attack and are also less likely to suffer from depression, schizophrenia, ADD/HD, autism, or Alzheimer's disease. It is estimated that only 40 percent of Americans consume an adequate supply of omega-3 fatty acids, and this national deficiency is reflected in our rising costs of health care.

Meat, poultry, eggs, and dairy products from grassfed or pastured animals are among the richest known source of another good fat called conjugated linoleic acid, or CLA. Animals raised exclusively on grass contain from three to five times more CLA than those raised on grains. Much of the CLA is stored in the fat of the animals and that is why including the fats from these animals in our diet is of great benefit to our health.

There is evidence that CLA may be a potent defense against cancer. In a Finnish study, women who had the highest levels of CLA in their diet had a 60 percent lower risk of breast cancer than those with the lowest CLA levels. We can all take advantage of this lowered risk simply by including one glass of raw or pastured milk, one or two ounces of grassfed cheese, or a small portion of grassfed meat in our daily diet. *It's that simple.*

In addition to CLA, other important vitamins accumulate in the fat of grassfed ruminants. In 1945, Dr. Weston A. Price described what he called "activator X" as a critical nutrient for optimal health. This "X-Factor" has now been identified as vitamin K_2, which accumulates in the ruminants' fat. K_2 is essential in helping our bones absorb vitamin D, a vitamin that many Americans are deficient in today and that I discuss in more depth below. Even vegetarians can benefit from grassfed cattle—butter from grassfed cows contains not only CLA but also the fat-soluble vitamins A, D, and E, and the "X-Factor" K_2.

GRASSFED, PASTURED, AND VITAMIN D

In *Primal Body, Primal Mind,* Nora Gedgaudas suggests that vitamin D could be the single most important vitamin for our overall health and is probably the most important antioxidant in the body. Vitamin D lowers the risk of all cancers, including skin cancers. It boosts the immune system and helps prevent autoimmune diseases like multiple sclerosis and rheumatoid arthritis, prevents cardiovascular disease, Parkinson's disease, and both type 1 and type 2 diabetes. Vitamin D also supports healthy brain function and moods and prevents seasonal affective disorder.

Vitamin D is found almost exclusively in the flesh and fats of grassfed animals and wild-caught fish. The diet of our ancestors included up to 4,000 IU or more of vitamin D daily. Today, the recommended daily allowance (RDA) is only 400 IU, which is completely inadequate to meet all the cellular requirements of maintaining our health. Though we can get vitamin D synthetically, simply taking a vitamin supplement is not as straightforward as we once thought. According to Nora, "What is referred to broadly as vitamin D is also found in the body in different forms. . . . A growing, very real problem is the excessive 'fortification' of processed foods with vitamin D as a means of marketing and selling. . . . This is a potentially great cause for concern and could lead to toxic and even immunosuppressive effects in people who consume vitamin D in excess. . . . The safest means of obtaining vitamin D is through exposure to sunlight" (pages 89–92). We need the natural vitamin D that only sunlight and animal sources (animals exposed to sunlight and a diet of grass) can provide.

Eggs from pastured hens are also far richer in vitamin D: when hens are raised out of doors and on a natural diet of bugs, seeds, vegetation, and sunlight exposure, their eggs have from three to six times more vitamin D than hens raised in confinement. Eating just two pastured eggs a day will give you anywhere from 63 to 126 percent of the daily recommended intake of vitamin D. The tricky part here is that the labeling of eggs in supermarkets is increasingly deceptive. Just because the label says "certified organic feed" or "all vegetarian diet" does not mean the chickens were pastured and allowed out of doors. You can ask your grocer if their store will carry pastured eggs, or you can find a local source. You can usually find pastured eggs at farmers' markets, though they are often more expensive. The best thing is to raise your own chickens.

Unfortunately some products are marketed as grassfed when they are not *entirely* grassfed. The American Grassfed Association is pushing hard for strict U.S. Department of Agriculture marketing guidelines. In the near future consumers will be able to purchase products that are certified and identifiable by the American Grassfed Association logo. In the meantime, you can ask for exclusively grassfed—*no grain finishing at all*—when purchasing these products. Talk to your local farmers' market producer about the way his or her animals are raised. Ask the person at your local meat counter to provide exclusively grassfed meat and pastured poultry. Be proactive! You can assist in bringing this awareness to your community and local grocery store. Refer to the Resources section at the back of the book for sources of grassfed and pastured meat and dairy products.

HUMANELY RAISED PORK

The current method of raising pork, in massive and inhumane feedlots, has brought on a new level of pollution in our country. The American industrial pork business is responsible for thousands of toxic-disease breeding grounds around the country. Pigs produce a huge amount of waste, and the reservoirs of this waste leach in to our waterways and coastal estuaries, causing massive algae blooms that deoxygenate the waters and kill millions of fish. The ponds of pig waste also evaporate noxious compounds into the air.

A recent news report on the inhumane treatment of piglets was so disturbing and severe that I will never buy commercially raised pork products again. I felt so badly about it that I had initially decided not to put any recipes with pork in this book. Fortunately, however, there are humane pork producers in the United States. I recommend you find one in your area. You can use the Humane Farm Animal Care organization and their Certified Humane website (www.hfaco .convio.net) to find a list of all the humane producers. *Certified Humane* means that the program meets certain standards, which include nutritious diet without antibiotics or hormones, and the animals are raised with shelter, resting areas, sufficient space, and the ability to engage in natural behaviors.

To see an example of what humanely raised pork should be, I invite you to go to the Beeler's Pork Farm website (www.beelerspurepork.com). I have purchased many of their pork products, which include ham, cheddar bratworst, bacon, sausage links, Italian sausage, and wieners. Beeler's pork products are also gluten-free with no fillers. Another California producer of humanely raised pork is Llano Seco Farm in Chico. They carry ham, bacon, spicy Andouille sausage, and fresh pork roasts, ribs, and chops.

SEAFOOD, TURNING THE TIDE

Ocean life today is threatened like no other time in our evolutionary history. Nothing is stripping our oceans of our critical supply of a high-quality protein source more than our current methods of corporate commercial fishing. The global catch of wild fish and the health of ocean ecosystems are now in severe decline. This situation, along with major oil spills, global warming, and radiation leakage from Fukoshima, is alarming. A severe decline in seafood will mean global famine. All countries on Earth must participate in preserving our oceans with sustainable fishing practices and safe management of our oceans.

Recently, farmed fish has overtaken the market as the leading source of seafood in the human diet, yet aquaculture is problematic and may also contribute to the decline in ocean health. Fish farming means that fish are grown in open pens, much like cattle feedlots. The pens are awash in excrement, which escapes and mixes with seawater. In order to combat these unsanitary conditions the fish are fed antibiotics, which also get into the oceans and subsequently into our bodies. The reason we are so resistant to current antibiotics is that they have leached into our food supply. The farmed fish are fed fishmeal, which may contain toxic substances such as PCBs.

IN SEARCH OF SUSTAINABLE SOLUTIONS

Today there is beginning to be consensus on the need for global standards and regulations regarding responsible fish-farming practices. As part of this effort, numerous conservation groups and advocates for healthy oceans have launched education and awareness programs to help educate consumers about marine health and sustainabilty.

The Monterey Bay Aquarium, for instance, launched a special exhibition called *Fishing for Solutions: What's the Catch?* The exhibition addressed the issues of inadequate fisheries' management, overfishing, bycatch, destruction of marine habitats by fishing gear and aquaculture operations, and skyrocketing demand for seafood from a larger, more affluent global population. Though this particular exhibit is no longer on display, the information is still available—along with many current updates on the topic—at the aquarium's website, which I invite you to visit: www.montereybayaquarium.org.

The Seafood Choice Alliance is an international association that advances the market for sustainable seafood. The alliance assists the seafood industry—including fishermen, fish farmers, distributors, wholesalers, retailers, and restaurants—making the marketplace economically, environmentally, and socially sustainable. Seafood Alliance has been inviting and challenging those corporations involved in mass-scale fishing operations to engage in more responsible behavior. They are encouraging a global solution to the threats facing our oceans.

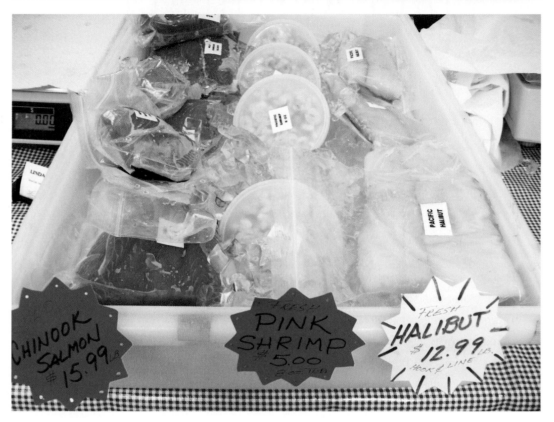

As responsible consumers we can now be more active in choosing sustainability at the fish counter when we shop. Conservation organizations, including Blue Ocean Institute, the Monterey Bay Aquarium Seafood Watch Program, and the Environmental Defense Fund, have developed "wallet cards" to guide our choices of sustainable seafoods. The wallet cards are generally categorized in a system of green for best choices, yellow for good choices, and red for endangered species to avoid. Another tool for consumers is Blue Ocean Institute's "Fish Phone," a sustainable seafood text-messaging service. Now consumers with a question about the origins of particular fish can send a text message with the name of the fish in question and rapidly get a response, along with alternative choices. Contact information for these organizations is found in the Resources section (page 258).

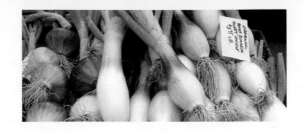

DIET AND HEALTH

It stands to reason that the more symptoms a person has physically, cognitively, or psychologically, the more primitive a diet (in other words, pre-agricultural or "primal") he or she ought to consider adopting to reclaim rightful health.

NORA GEDGAUDAS

GLUTEN, THE CULPRIT FOR SO MANY ILLS

There's a rarely suspected, underlying culprit in grains that is wreaking havoc on our national health in epidemic proportions. *It is gluten.* Gluten is found in many grains that we typically consume, such as durum, semolina, graham, spelt, kamut, triticale, rye, barley, and even oats. Also, genetic changes to our American strains of wheat, which give them higher gluten content than European strains, have significantly exacerbated the problem. Due to this there's a marked increase in the incidence of full-blown celiac disease in the United States. Celiac disease is the extreme malabsorption of nutrients, which leads to many other diseases.

According to Nora Gedgaudas, "Gluten can affect all organ systems (including your brain, heart, and kidneys), your extended nervous system, your moods, your immunological functioning, your digestive system, and even your musculoskeletal system—truly almost all of you, from your hair follicles down to your toenails and everything in between" (page 34).

Due to our increasing deterioration of health, we and our children are now extremely sensitive to grains, legumes, starch, milk (casein), sugar, and most all processed foods, which are likely to have hidden gluten in the ingredients. In addition to being used as an additive and stabilizing agent in processed foods, gluten is also in pharmaceuticals and health care products like shampoos and lotions.

Perhaps you may not know you are gluten sensitive. Undiagnosed gluten sensitivity can cause many serious health problems, ruin the quality of your life, and even cause death, so it's wise to be tested. Don't guess about your problem. Work with a physician or a licensed health care professional who can guide you to a test lab such as Cyrex Labs. Gluten sensitivity can lead to brain and mood disorders (broken brains), irritable and inflamed bowels, autoimmune diseases, heart problems, and even cancer. Sometimes the symptoms are delayed (for days or months), so you won't necessarily tie them to gluten consumption. As Nora points out, "Grains are rarely suspected as the original culprit, though every one of these disorders, among many more, can be traced to often insidious gluten intolerance. Gluten sensitivity is rarely obvious to the afflicted, and many people are even entirely surprised to learn they have this sensitivity. I know I was"* (page 43).

A gluten-free diet will require a completely new approach to eating that will affect a person's entire life. People with celiac disease have to be extremely careful about what they buy for lunch at school or work, eat at cocktail parties, or grab from the refrigerator for a midnight snack. Dining out can be challenging, even dangerous, as the person with celiac disease must learn how to scrutinize the menu for foods with gluten and question the waiter about possible hidden sources. Cross-contamination is always possible, and even trace amounts of gluten will trigger a reaction that may last for months. Even a trace (0.03 percent) of gluten in a food product can cause a reaction for a gluten-sensitive individual. It's just not worth the risk. *Avoidance of gluten must be 100 percent.*

Remember that just because a label says gluten-free or organic does not mean that it is necessarily healthy for you. Nothing could be further from the truth. Many gluten-free and organic products contain contaminated grains, bad oils, and high sugar content. Beware of junk food masquerading as healthy. Nutritional power bars are some of the worst offenders because of their grain and high sugar content. Plus they are expensive. Gluten intolerance and carbohydrate intolerance normally go hand in hand.

Even foods that are frequent substitutions for gluten may cause food sensitivities and problems. You may be very surprised to learn that even when you remove gluten from the diet, it may not be sufficient to restore full intestinal health. Other grains such as rice, quinoa, corn, soy, and buckwheat, which are commonly substituted for gluten, may still cause gut inflammation (IBS) and other hard-to-identify symptoms.

---

*For an in-depth examination of the dangers of gluten consumption and all of the allergic reactions it causes in the body, see chapter 3, "Grains, Are they Really a Health Food?" in *Primal Body, Primal Mind*.

Nora makes a point of saying, "As there is no human dietary grain requirement—and since grain consumption causes so many known health problems due to its anti-nutrient content, its tryptophan-poor profile, high omega-6 levels, and its mainly starch-based content, as well as its allergy and sensitivity potential—there is little reason to include grains in the diet of anyone seeking optimal health. In fact, the fewer grains consumed the better. Zero is by far the best" (page 30).

THE MILK DEVIL, *CASEIN*

There is growing concern about another problem substance found in milk that is causing just as many ills as gluten: casein. Casein, a protein, can have two forms, A1 or A2. All milk was once A2 until a genetic mutation—which occurred anywhere from five to ten thousand years ago—affected some strains of European cattle. This mutation changed the original A2 protein by one single amino acid, resulting in the A1 strain. This "milk devil" is called by different names, including A1 beta-casein, and beta-caseomorphin-7, or BMC7 for short.

As is the case with gluten, our bodies have not genetically adapted to this new strain of A1 milk, thus creating a host of health problems. While it is beyond the scope of this book to address all the health ramifications of A1 beta-casein, it is important to note that it has now been implicated in many illnesses, including heart disease, type 1 diabetes, autism, and schizophrenia.

There is evidence suggesting that the milk devil (A1 beta-casein) is produced only by cows that originated in northern Europe and then from only some of these cows. The first population of cows arrived in the United States from Europe around 1783, and it was only by accident that some of these cows were the mutated A1 strain. Apparently Asian, African, and some southern European cattle are free of the mutation and are still A2. In the United States, Canada, New Zealand, Australia, and northern Europe, the majority of the cows produce A1 milk. Anyone consuming milk in the United States can be sure they are getting high levels of A1 casein in their milk.

I suggest reading the extremely well-researched and informative book *Devil in the Milk; Illness, Health, and the Politics of A1 and A2 Milk* by Keith Woodford, particularly if you have a child with autism or if you happen to be casein intolerant, as I recently found out. You may well want to consider avoiding cow's milk and products made from cow's milk, especially if you or your children are symptomatic. Just as with gluten sensitivity, symptoms can vary and also be delayed, so you may not necessarily tie them to casein intolerance. Beyond that, the book provides compelling evidence that we should switch our herds of cows back over to the A2 strain. This would be a monumental undertaking that would require the complete support of our national dairy interests.

It must be noted that goats, sheep, yaks, and humans produce only A2 milk. However, even milk from sheep and goats contains casein. Currently there are no tests for casein sensitivity to sheep or goat's milk. Some individuals will have a reaction to all casein regardless of the animal, while others may only react to a certain mammal's milk. The amino acid chains differ from species to species, so this gives the opportunity for some people to be able to tolerate casein from one type of animal over another. At this time, the only way to determine whether a person has a reaction to goat or sheep's milk is to conduct a challenge test. It is recommended to be totally casein free for a minimum of six months prior to doing this test.

Primal Body, Primal Mind warns that there is also "a potent cross-reactivity to casein that has additionally been demonstrated to be similar to an immunologic reactivity to gluten" (page 37). Apparently a similar inflammatory response to that of gluten also occurs in about 50 percent of the patients with celiac disease. Nora's chapter "Grains: Are They Really a Health Food?" provides a list of the most common *true* potentially cross-reactive compounds. (You may also go to the Cyrex Lab website to see this list and read more about cross-reactivity at www .cyrexlabs.com.) She points out that

> casein is among the most common co-sensitive agents with gluten, but the immune system can come to react to almost anything if gluten consumption persists. Cross-reactivity, which is the tendency to react to substances either genetically or structurally similar to gluten or that our immune system has merely to associate with gluten, is an added concern for many. This can be a very real and frustrating problem. Once multiple food sensitivities take over, they can cause a vicious cycle that worsens with time and becomes extremely difficult to correct. Autoimmune processes—often multiple ones—can be a very common result." (page 38)

In some of the recipes I have included raw milk substitutions for pasteurized milk products from commercially raised cows, sheep, or goats. However, *do be aware of casein sensitivity!* Don't assume you *don't* have food sensitivities just because you are not experiencing symptoms. The only way to be sure is to be tested.

THE TRUTH ABOUT RAW AND PROCESSED MILK

Our ancestors ate everything raw for millions of years, and we *evolved* on raw food. "Raw" (unpasteurized) milk is nature's perfect food. For generations, traditional societies thrived consuming the raw milk, cream, nutrient-rich butter, and cheeses from their grassfed herds of cows, sheep, and goats. These animals were also free of hormones, antibiotics, and pesticides (which today are found in supplemented grain feed). If raw milk had been dangerous we wouldn't be here today.* Raw milk, cream, and butter also contain the "Wulzen factor," a compound discovered by researcher Rosalind Wulzen that is potentially beneficial for healthy joints as well as protecting against hardening of the arteries, cataracts, and calcification of the pineal gland.

Highly processed pasteurized and ultra-pasteurized milk products contain rancid fats and oxidized cholesterol and are likely to aggravate casein-related food sensitivities. The "low-fat" and "non-fat" milks are high in carbohydrates. Powdered milk, which contains large amounts of oxidized cholesterol, is added to skim milk and 1- and 2-percent milk products to give them body and texture. Heavy cream, on the other hand, is essentially all fat, with no carbohydrates.

AVOIDING rBGH

Recombinant bovine growth hormone (rBGH) is a synthetic (man-made) hormone used by some dairy farmers to increase milk production in cows. It has been used in the United States since it was approved by the FDA in 1993. According to the Organic Consumers Association there are many reasons to avoid dairy products with rBGH. Following is a list of the major health concerns related to rBGh, taken with permission from the book *What's in Your Milk?* by Dr. Samual S. Epstein.

- rBGH makes cows sick. Monsanto (the makers of the synthetic hormone

---

*If you are concerned about the safety of raw milk please visit the Real Milk website at http.realmilk .com/appeal-jun06-testimonials.html.

POSILAC) has been forced to admit to about 20 toxic effects.*

- rBGH milk is contaminated by pus, due to the mastitis commonly induced by rBGH, and antibiotics used to treat the mastitis.
- rBGH milk is chemically and nutritionally different from natural milk.
- rBGH milk is contaminated with rBGH, traces of which are absorbed in the gut.
- rBGH is supercharged with high levels of a natural growth factor (IGF-1), which is readily absorbed into the gut. Excess levels of IGF-1 have been incriminated as a cause of breast, colon, and prostate cancers. IGF-1 blocks natural defense mechanisms against early submicroscopic cancers.
- rBGH milk consumers . . . are at a high risk for cancer.
- rBGH factory farms pose a major threat to the viability of small dairy farms.
- rBGH enriches Monsanto while posing dangers, without any benefits, to consumers, especially in view of the current national surplus of milk.

Nowadays many milk producers have removed rBGH from their milk products. This must be stated on the label, so watch for it. If you're not able to find any rBGH-free products, you can refer to the Organic Consumers Association website (www.organicconsumers.org), which lists the top rBGH and rBGH-free processors.

ANTIBIOTICS IN OUR FOOD SUPPLY AND CONSUMER LABELS

The overuse of antibiotics in farm animals and farmed fish is creating antibiotic resistance in the human population, which means antibiotics will cease working to cure us when we most need them. Also, these antibiotics kill the beneficial microbes in our gut, opening the door for pathogenic bacteria and an overpopulation of yeasts, which in turn negatively affects our immune system. As consumers, we must demand that food products be produced in a way that antibiotics are not necessary. We can assume that commercially raised animals have high levels of antibiotics in their meat and milk. The grains these animals are fed cause inflammation in their intestines, which is why they are fed antibiotics. *All the more reason to buy grassfed only.*

---

*Elanco, a division of Eli Lilly and Company now makes POSILAC.

Two ways we can reduce the use of antibiotics in commercial feeding operations (CFOs) is by first educating the public and second by demanding accurate labeling standards. Labeling is the key to distinguishing "alternative" animal production practices from the current "conventional" practices that involve heavy and routine administration of antibiotics. Claims and standards must be made clear and relevant to consumers. Labeling that *intends to obscure* important differences between conventional and alternative production systems will deny customers true disclosure. We all have a right to *the freedom to discern and choose* between the products from these different kinds of systems. In addition, unclear label claims undercut the ability of alternative producers to fairly compete for customers by making it harder for these producers to differentiate their products. Fraudulent claims put at risk the livelihoods of farmers who have staked their financial futures on raising animals without the use of antibiotics. We must be diligent in protecting the public health even if our government is not.

CUMULATIVE CARBOHYDRATE CONSUMPTION

After reading *The Schwarzbein Principle, The UltraMind Solution,* and *Primal Body, Primal Mind,* I have become convinced that our *cumulative carbohydrate consumption* in the United States is the cause of many diseases. Primary among them are hypoglycemia and type 2 diabetes. Nora Gedgaudas describes hypoglycemia as the result of cells using available glucose so rapidly that the blood cannot readily meet the constant demand for more fuel. The cells actually become starved. Glucose deficiency drastically alters brain function, because the brain cells cannot store glucose and require a continuous supply of glucose to generate energy. In a state of glucose starvation, the brain can no longer direct vital processes, disrupting physical and emotional behavior. Mental symptoms frequently resulting from hypoglycemia include:

- anxiety
- headaches
- fatigue
- irritability
- nervousness
- depression
- crying spells

- confusion or forgetfulness
- insomnia
- phobias and fears
- disruptive outbursts
- dis-perceptions (perceiving something inaccurately)
- dizziness, vertigo, faintness
- low blood pressure
- cold hands and feet

As mentioned earlier, according to Dr. Hyman, our "brains are broken" because of our body's allergic reaction to gluten and other toxic substances that we are ingesting. Chronic carbohydrate consumption, in general, depletes serotonin in the body and brain. It also depletes the B vitamins necessary to convert amino acids into essential neurotransmitters for brain function. *Our children and their developing brains are especially vulnerable.*

The Center for Disease Control estimates that if current dietary habits persist, as many as one-third of our nation's children will become diabetic. The major cause is a form of malnutrition tied to highly processed, prepackaged, and fast foods that are high in refined sugar and trans-fats and short on vitamins and complex carbohydrates. Children are much more intolerant than adults of grains and legumes, starch, milk, and sugars (including honey, maple syrup, agave, and fruit juices). The national cost of caring for tens of millions of type-2 diabetics is draining public coffers and personal wealth.

Worldwide diabetes has now reached pandemic proportions and continues to be on the increase. According to the American Diabetes Association, diabetes now affects close to twenty million people in the United States, and there are also twenty million pre-diabetics at risk. The same is true in Europe, India, and China. If the current trend continues it is estimated that one in three children born after 2000 will have diabetes. At the turn of the twentieth century this figure was less than one in a hundred.

Many people still believe that a lifetime of medication is the only solution to diabetes and that it is incurable once you have it. But diabetes can be cured by a change in diet that, among other factors, includes eliminating grains and sugars. All commercially made cookies, crackers, pies, cakes, and pastries should be completely avoided, even if they say "organic" or "gluten-free." It's very difficult to break the habit of eating these foods (if you can even call them foods), because we are so much in the habit of continually treating ourselves to sugar and carbohydrates when under stress. But these high-carb foods actually increase stress.

Of all addictions, including addiction to alcohol and other drugs, sugar is one of the toughest to quit. I know from experience. It has taken me most of a lifetime to break this habit, and I sympathize with everyone who has to face it. But *now* is the time to do it. You can do it if you *clean house* and only have "safe" foods at home. You do not want to raise children who are addicted to sugar and refined carbohydrates. It's now highly probable that autism, ADD, and ADHD are caused or exacerbated by sugar, refined carbohydrates, gluten, casein, and food allergies. Why put our children at risk?

The research is in, the scientific papers have been written and published, and now the facts are known. We can no longer say we didn't have the correct information. Nora Gedgaudas firmly suggests that "the closer you can come to eliminating all forms of sugar and starch (including grains, bread, pasta, rice, potatoes, desserts, juices, alcohol, honey, maple syrup. . . , etc.) by far the better" (page 301).

This book is meant to be a transition to a healthier, energy-enhancing way of eating. I leave it up to you to read and then to test what these experts are saying by implementing the Paleo diet of our ancestors.

CHILDREN DO NOT HAVE TO BE OVERWEIGHT, BUT THEY DO NEED HEALTHY FATS!

Dr. Diana Schwarzbein, founder of the Endocrinology Institute of Santa Barbara, reminds us in her book *The Schwarzbein Principle* that we have moved further away from the diet of our ancestors by feeding our children processed junk foods. It is a common practice of food manufacturers to remove the fats from these food products and then to add harmful chemicals or more sugar to add flavor.

According to Dr. Schwarzbein, "Processed foods are fattening, first, because they contain sugar, which raises insulin levels and, second, because they instigate the vicious cycle of carbohydrate craving. This is why many children are overweight today. *To make matters worse, children now eat low-fat foods.* Unfortunately, we have been taught to worry more about the fat content than the chemical and sugar content of these foods. We've been led to believe that, as long as there is little or no fat, we are doing no harm" (page 195).

Dr. Schwarzbein also states that "adults need fat in their diet to replenish and nourish the body, but children need fat even more to develop into healthy adults. Healthful fats in foods are the source of the fat-soluble vitamins A, E, D, and K. Taking vitamin supplements has not shown the same health benefits as eating these good fats that contain the fat-soluble vitamins. . . . When children come to me for 'genetic obesity,' I immediately switch them to a balanced diet sufficient in proteins and fats while decreasing their carbohydrate consumption. Every one of these children loses body fat and gains her or his ideal body composition" (pages 195, 197).

THE HEALTH RISKS OF GMOS
(GENETICALLY MODIFIED ORGANISMS)

Since 1996 Americans, without their full knowledge and consent, have been eating genetically modified ingredients in most of their processed food. Genetically modified plants, such as soybeans, corn, cottonseed, and canola have foreign genes forced into their DNA. The inserted genes come from bacteria and viruses that have never before been in the human food supply. Gene insertion is done by shooting genes from a "gene gun" into a plate of cells or by introducing bacteria with foreign DNA into the cell. The altered cell is then cloned into the plant. These processes create massive collateral damage, causing mutations in hundreds or thousands of locations throughout the plant's DNA. Natural genes can be deleted or permanently turned on or off, and hundreds may change their levels of expression.

At the very least, these foods should bear a "WARNING" label, because genetically modified organisms have not been tested for safety and have already been linked to serious toxic and allergic reactions in humans and livestock. The inserted gene, which is often rearranged, may transfer from the food into our body's cells or into the DNA of bacteria inside of us. The genetically modified protein produced by the gene may have unintended properties or effects on the human genome.

The primary reason GMOs were designed in the first place was to make them tolerant to herbicides, thus increasing crop productivity and reducing world famine. However, increased crop yield has not happened. The major producer of herbicides and genetically engineered seeds is Monsanto. The four major GM plants—soy, corn, canola, and cotton—are designed to survive an otherwise deadly dose of weed killer. As a result all these crops have a much higher residue of toxic herbicides, and we should avoid consuming them for that reason alone. Many genetically modified plants also have a *built-in pesticide*. A gene from the soil bacterium *Bacillus thuringiensis* (Bt) is inserted into the plant's DNA, where it secretes the insect-killing Bt toxin in every cell. *You cannot wash the herbicides and pesticides off these foods. They are literally part of the plant.* This is very disturbing, especially when you consider feeding these altered foods to children.

Also, it is now suspected that one of the reasons for bee colony collapse is the result of bees ingesting the built-in pesticide in the plant's nectar. The toxin either poisons the bee or interferes with its navigation system, impairing its ability to fly back to the hive. This is just one of the reasons these plants should be made illegal. California's trillion dollar agricultural economy is dependent on bee pollination. GM plants are not worth the risk.

About 68 percent of GM crops are herbicide tolerant, about 19 percent of crops produce their own pesticide, and another 13 percent produce a pesticide and are herbicide tolerant. Once aware of these dangers no one in their right mind would continue to consume these plants. Yet, *the FDA does not require any safety evaluations for GMOs.* Why isn't the FDA protecting us? Since 1992 the FDA has claimed that there is no risk in eating GMOs and that these foods are not substantially different from conventionally grown foods. Still some FDA scientists have warned that GMOs could potentially create unpredictable, hard-to-detect side effects, including allergies, toxins, new diseases, and nutritional deficiencies. Long-term safety studies have been recommended but never done.

Nonprofit organizations are stepping in to fill the gap. The Institute for Responsible Technology website given in the Resources section (page 260) is a good source for information on GMOs. In addition, the Center for Food Safety is seeking to halt the approval, commercialization, or release of any new genetically engineered crops until they have been proved safe for human consumption and the environment.

All of us must demand that Congress pass laws requiring clear labels on food products that contain genetically engineered ingredients. We must also seek to limit and reduce the proliferation of genetically engineered crops.

FOOD ADDITIVES TO AVOID

If it doesn't look like food, it probably isn't! We have to educate ourselves about food additives, because the FDA still allows many harmful and potentially deadly substances to be added to our national food supply. This has to stop, and it's time we took matters back into our own hands. Trying to be heard in Congress over all the food-manufacturing lobbyists, commercial agribusiness interests, and petrochemical fertilizer companies is going to be really slow going. Our *vote* to have unadulterated whole foods begins in our local communities, at our farmers' markets and grocery stores. *Read food labels!* Don't buy the bad stuff and maybe all the manufacturers and *pushers of toxic food ingredients* will get the message. Be an activist and let them know we're mad as hell and we're not going to eat it any more.

In addition to the recommendations already made, the most important things to avoid fall into four major categories: preservatives, other dangerous ingredients, nutrient-poor foods, and unhealthy beverages.

Preservatives

Preservatives are additives in food that help keep food from spoiling. Unfortunately many of these substances are highly toxic and can cause allergic reactions, illness, and even death. The Food Allergen Labeling and Consumer Protection Act of 2004 requires food manufacturers to disclose the eight most common allergens on the labels of packaged foods. However, this is not very well monitored. Also, the manufacturers do not have to disclose an ingredient until a certain percentage is present in the food. Even trace amounts of a toxin can be devastating to a sensitive individual. Why risk public health unnecessarily? We need to be informed and *very* vigilant on the topic of food additives, especially in order to protect our children and their developing brains.

> **Benzoic acid (or sodium benzoate)** is added to margarine, fruit juices, and carbonated beverages. It has been known to cause severe allergic reactions and death.
>
> **Nitrates** are used to preserve meats and are found in lunchmeats, ham, and bacon products. Nitrates can cause asthma, nausea, vomiting, and headaches.
>
> **Sodium nitrite** is capable of being converted to nitrous acid when ingested. Even though animal testing has shown that nitrous acid causes high rates of cancer in animals, it is still in use.
>
> **Sulfites** (which are found in wines) can also cause some of the same symptoms as nitrates. Sulfites are used to prevent fungal spoilage, as well as browning, which occurs on fruits and vegetables.

Sulfur dioxide is a toxin used to preserve dried fruits and molasses. It is used to prevent brown spots on fresh fruits and vegetables such as apples and potatoes. Sulfur dioxide bleaches out rot, hiding inferior fruits and vegetables and destroying the B vitamins in produce.

Other Dangerous Ingredients

Aside from preservatives there are other additives and ingredients that you should be particularly wary of. The following is a short list of the most prevalent additives and ingredients, which can be found in most processed foods. Avoiding processed foods altogether is a huge step you can take toward good health.

Agave is a newly touted popular sweetener, but it is just as glycating and even more concentrated in damaging fructose than high fructose corn syrup (see below). It is 70 percent to 90 percent pure fructose!

Artificial flavors have been linked to allergic reactions and behavioral problems. There are more than 200 of them in use. These flavorings are not required to be listed in detail because the Food and Drug Administration recognizes them as safe.

Artificial sweeteners such as saccharine and aspartame have been linked to behavioral problems, hyperactivity, and allergies. Saccharin has been shown to increase bladder cancer in animal testing and is therefore required to carry a warning label.

Bleach (oxides of nitrogen, chlorine, chloride, nitrosyl, and benzoyl peroxide), mixed with a wide variety of chemical salts, is used to process wheat into commercial baked goods. Chloride oxide, which catalyzes a chemical reaction that destroys beta cells in the pancreas, is now being linked to diabetes. Even though the toxicity of chloride oxide is recognized, the FDA still allows its use.

High fructose corn syrup is *deadly*. This ingredient, used in many prepackaged food products, beverages, and condiments, is manufactured using genetically modified corn and a plethora of nasty synthetic chemicals.

Monosodium glutamate had been banned in baby food, but now it is back. Processed *free glutamic acid,* the reactive component in monosodium glutamate, is known to be toxic to the nervous system. Synthetic MSG (AuxiGro WP Plant Metabolic Primer, manufactured by Emerald Bio Agriculture) is now being sprayed on all kinds of crops, such as fruits, nuts, vegetables, and grains. These crops are then *used in baby food,* as well as being in wide use in other food products as well. As yet no one knows what the long-terms effects of this substance are, which is one more reason to buy organic produce only.

Emulsifiers, stabilizers, and thickeners are included in many processed foods. Propylene glycol, for example, is a synthetic solvent, which is recognized as toxic to the skin and also considered to be a neurological toxicant. The Food and Drug Administration still deems it to be safe. Many vitamins contain this ingredient, so watch out for it.

High salt content in the form of refined sodium chloride is a common ingredient in processed foods. Sodium is added to fast foods and even sodas (it makes you even thirstier so you drink more).

Hydrogenated or partially hydrogenated oils appear in most prepackaged foods and bottled salad dressings. All commercial canola and soybean oils are also partially hydrogenated as part of the deodorization process and should *never* be consumed. *Avoid all artificial trans-fats and rancid fats.*

Propylene oxide gas (PPO), a known carcinogen, is sometimes used to sterilize nuts. Be sure not to buy any nuts that have been treated with this chemical, which is toxic and poisonous. The European Union has prohibited the use of PPO on any human food product. The USDA and FDA still allow it. Inquire at your store if their fruits and nuts have been exposed to PPO.

Sugars: It is not enough to avoid refined sugar and high fructose corn syrup. For optimum health, you also need to avoid *naturally occurring sugars such as honey, maple syrup, and dried fruit.* Read labels for sugar content. It all adds up to being overweight and diabetic.

Nutrient-Poor Foods

Certain foods should be avoided by everyone who wishes to experience optimum health. In addition, each person needs to pay attention to their own particular food allergies and eliminate those foods from his or her diet. If you haven't been tested, the following is a short list of foods to which many people experience sensitivity: grains in general, dairy (casein), soy, nuts, eggs, and the "nightshade" plants like tomatoes, potatoes, and eggplant. A good resource for further investigation is chapter 28, "What About Food Allergies and Sensitivities?" in *Primal Body, Primal Mind.* In addition to the foods specifically listed below, it is prudent to also avoid the following: low- or no-fiber foods (a high-fiber diet is essential for good health), and legumes and grains, as both contain more starch than protein. They also contain high levels of phytic acid, which actively binds minerals and eliminates them from the body.

Commercial Dairy Products: Almost all dairy cows today (85–95%) are raised in confinement on a diet of grain, mostly corn. This is the agribusiness method because it's efficient and cost effective. The grain-based diet causes pH changes in the cows and increases the need for the use of antibiotics. The result is that the omega-3 fatty acids in grain-fed cows are very low, and the omega-6 fatty acids, which most people are consuming too many of these days, are high. Low-fat dairy products (skim milk, 1%, and 2%) are made up mainly of carbohydrates and should be avoided. (*Heavy cream has no carbohydrates.*) The low-fat milks also contain large amounts of oxidized cholesterol. Conventional dairy products, such as cheese spreads, dips, and ice creams may also contain gluten as an additive in the form of vegetable gum or modified food starch. Read labels carefully.

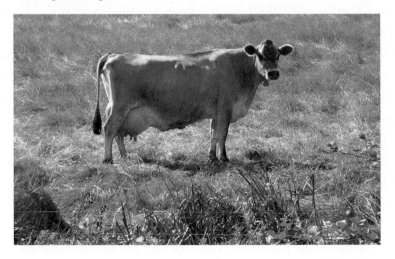

Soy Alert!: The Weston A. Price Foundation is a nonprofit nutrition education foundation dedicated to restoring nutrient-dense foods to the human diet through education, research, and activism. The foundation is spearheading a national campaign to warn consumers about the dangers of modern soy foods. Their efforts are congruent with the warning given by Nora Gedgaudas in *Primal Body, Primal Mind*.

Contrary to popular belief, soy (particularly tofu, soy milk, and soy protein isolate) is among the newest additions to the human diet. Soy has been considered unfit for human consumption since ancient times, but chemical processing methods created by corporate interests have created an "all-new" soy, purported to be the cornerstone of health and longevity. The unsuspecting public has unfortunately succumbed to misleading claims and other marketing ploys to increasingly seek out meat substitutes, including texturized vegetable protein (also called TVP), tofu, soy milk, and soy protein powders. Many have been led to believe that these foods somehow prevent cancer and heart disease and can provide quality protein in their diets. Nothing could be further from the truth. (page 49)

For these reasons you will not find soy as an ingredient in this book. Instead I have replaced tamari or soy sauce with Coconut Secret Raw Aminos, which are 100 percent gluten-free.

Bottled Salad Dressings should be completely eliminated. They may have a label that says "all natural," but most contain wheat and soy ingredients. Here are the listed ingredients on a salad dressing label I have right on my desk: "soybean oil, maltodextrin, sugar, salt, soy, modified food starch, soy lecithin, corn oil, carrageenan, phosphoric acid, artificial flavor, disodium phosphate, xanthan gum, monosodium glutamate, artificial color, disodium inosinate, disodium guanylate with sorbic acid, potassium sorbate and calcium disodium EDTA added as a preservatives." Yuk! Why would you want to eat that horrible stuff? Make your own homemade dressing and your salads will taste fabulous.

Refined Foods: White rice and refined flours, which are found in white breads, pasta, cookies, and numerous junk foods, are wreaking havoc with our health. With the brown husk of the grain removed, the remaining refined starches are broken down quickly into sugar and absorbed immediately into the blood stream, causing glucose levels to rise, thus increasing the risk of diabetes and obesity. Refining destroys most of the nutrients in the foods. Healthy unsaturated fatty acids are lost during the milling process. Vitamin E is significantly destroyed. Other nutrients such as vitamins and minerals are also lost.

Processed Luncheon Meats, Smoked Meats, and Sausages: All processed meats should also be removed from your refrigerator. Many of these products contain sodium nitrates, grain fillers (gluten again), artificial colorings, and flavors. You can purchase sausages with no grain fillers, such as Bruce Aidell's Organic Chicken Sausages. Amylu Chicken Sausages are entirely *gluten free* and pork-casing free. Your Thanksgiving turkey, if it is injected with a basting liquid, is probably toxic. Only buy pastured or organic turkeys. See producers in the Resources section (page 259).

Charcoal Grilled Food: There is evidence that charbroiled foods may increase the risk of cancer, so it is probably best to keep charcoal-grilled foods to a minimum.

Unhealthy Beverages

What we drink is just as important as what we eat. When it comes to beverages, we can assume that most commercial offerings are not healthy. Again, read the label. Look at the sugar content first and remember fructose *is* sugar. You definitely want to keep sodas out of your house if you have children; they are the number one contributor to obesity and diabetes.

Unfiltered Water: The importance of *pure water* in your diet cannot be overemphasized, especially for the health of your growing children. Our current water supplies in the United States have been exposed to fluoride, pesticides, pharmaceuticals (antibiotics are now in our water supply), heavy metals, harmful microbes, and other toxins. If you can avoid it do not buy water in plastic bottles, because the plastic contains toxic phthalates or bisphenol. Rather, I highly recommend that you use a water filter, such as a reverse osmosis filter, which can be installed in your home. Use your filtered water to cook with and to make coffee, iced teas, and other beverages that you and your family consume. See the Resources section (page 259) for reverse osmosis water filters, as well as contact information for a water-testing laboratory if you wish to have your water tested.

Other Beverages: Avoid all carbonated beverages, instant drinks, and drinks that are processed with additives, emulsifiers, and stabilizers. Do not buy instant coffees or teas, cocoa mixes with sugar and artificial flavorings, flavored malted milk, commercial chocolate milk, and ground coffees, which contain grains and artificial flavors. *Do not buy your children harmful beverages with high fructose corn syrup, agave, high fruit sugars, and artificial flavors and colors. All those ingredients are toxins that go through the blood-brain barrier and affect brain function.*

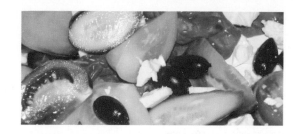

PALEO PANTRY: SETTING THE STAGE FOR SUCCESS

Make the kitchen your favorite room in the house so it will be a pleasure to prepare your meals. Include your favorite music to play while you cook. Organize your cooking tools attractively in containers that are handy to the stove. Have your good oils, sea salt assortment, and pepper grinder at hand as well. You are an artist. The ingredients are your artist's palette.

RECOMMENDED TOOLS
FOR THE PLEASURE OF COOKING

The right cooking tools will contribute to your overall success and add to your cooking enjoyment. Quality tools will last a lifetime if you take proper care of them. Here is my list of recommended tools:

- small kitchen scale
- instant-read meat thermometer
- candy thermometer (for making yogurt and kefir)
- good-quality knives (you don't need many): two sizes of chef's knives, a meat slicer, and a sharp paring knife
- small plastic cutting boards that can go in the dishwasher: various colors to distinguish those for meats and those for veggies
- large stainless steel stock pot with lid
- 2- and 4-quart stainless steel saucepans with lids (check out ceramic cookware too)

- 8- and 12-inch sauté pans (heavy-bottomed stainless steel)
- food processor
- blender or Vita-Mix
- coffee grinder for spices and seeds
- several sizes wire whisks
- non-meltable rubber spatulas
- assorted measuring cups and measuring spoons
- microplaners/graters for grating ginger and lemon zest
- 2 heavy stainless steel sheet pans
- 2 rectangular glass baking dishes, 9 × 13 inches
- 2 glass pie pans, 9 or 10 inch
- several sizes of fluted tart pans
- mortar and pestle
- nut milk bag (optional)

I do not recommend using microwave ovens for cooking. They are known to destroy the nutrient value of your food and also may lead to other potentially damaging effects.

STOCKING THE PANTRY

It's fun to stock your pantry with your favorite items that will inspire your cooking. I have suggested some of the following ingredients and products as a guide, but I'm sure you will add to this list. The main idea behind a well-stocked pantry is to support spur-of-the-minute creations.

Love
The most important ingredient for your pantry is love. Be sure to keep a lot of it on hand. It is our love of cooking and feeding our families and ourselves that is the true nourishment. Our bodies know when food is lovingly prepared, and love is the real fuel that helps us to embrace all of life's wonders and predicaments as well.

Essential Fats and Oils for Cooking
Good oils, like the ones listed below, should be the only ones you use when preparing food. Because oils are high in calories, you will need to determine the correct amount of daily oils for your individual body's requirements. *The freshness of the oils is of utmost importance.* It is also important to keep in mind that certain

oils, such as avocado oil, flax oil, and olive oil, should not be heated. They are for salad dressings or are to be used as "finishing" oils only.

Olive Oil

Olive oil is healthy for you and it's delicious. Not all olive oils are the same, however, and can vary in quality. The best method for harvesting olives is by hand. Olives tend to bruise when allowed to drop on the ground. Bruised olives may ferment and oxidize, which leads to an inferior quality oil. Of course, hand harvesting is labor intensive. The reason such care is necessary is because hand-picked olives produce a pure "extra virgin" oil.

California has become just as famous for its wonderful olive oils as it has for its award-winning wines. The five varieties of olives commonly grown in northern and central California are Arbequena, Ascalano, Frantoio, Manzanillo, and Mission. Some of the producers of premium olive oils are Bava Family Grove (Colline de Santa Cruz), Carriage Vineyards (Arbequena and Manzanillo Extra Virgin Olive Oil), Olivina Mission (Extra Virgin Unfiltered Olive Oil), McEvoy Ranch (Organic Extra Virgin Olive Oil), Lucero Flavored Olive Oils (great as a finishing oil), Robbins Family Farm Tuscan Blend, and B. R. Cohn, just to name a few. Bariani Stone Crushed organic olive oil is fabulous. Some of the common aromas and tastes found in certified California extra virgin olive oils are nutty, almond, grassy, fruity, floral, peppery, chili peppers, tomato, artichoke, apple, olives, butter, and caramel.

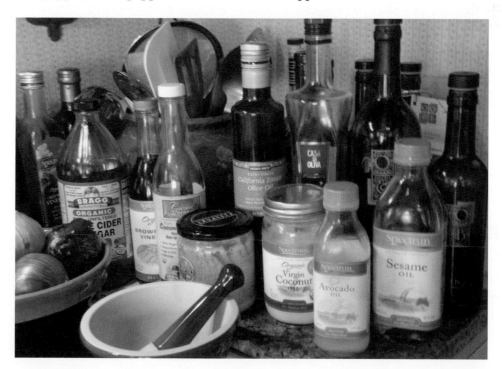

What about imported olive oils and inexpensive or discounted oils from the grocery store? Olive oil is perishable. Keep in mind that imported oils arrive months to years after production. The imported or discounted olive oils may have sat on a grocery store shelf and will have lost their freshness. These oils are more likely to taste rancid, bitter, metallic, musty, or smell fermented. Rancid oils are dangerous to consume, causing free-radicals.

Nut Oils

Nut oils can really spruce up your salads, vegetables, and seafood. Just a little of the oil can be drizzled on food for a truly wonderful taste sensation. One of the world's most famous producers of artisan nut oil is J. LeBlanc from Burgundy, France. This company has been in the nut oil business for 130 years. J. LeBlanc makes the oils in small batches, resulting in oils that taste exactly like the nuts from which they are made.

Organic Unrefined Virgin Coconut Oil and Coconut Butter

Virgin coconut oil has been used to cook with since ancient times. It has been used in the Ayurvedic medicine of India and has long been advocated for its thera-peutic qualities. Coconut oil contains no trans-fatty acids. It is a superb cooking oil because its chemical structure remains intact and is therefore resistant to the mutation of fatty acid chains even at high temperatures. Research shows that the medium chain fatty acids found in coconut oil boost the body's metabolism, raise body temperature, and help to provide energy necessary for weight loss. Coconut oil provides *satiation,* which is necessary for weight loss. If you use coconut oil on a consistent basis you provide vital nourishment to every cell of your body. Virgin coconut oil is rich in lauric acid (also found in mother's breast milk), a nutrient that supports the immune system. Lauric acid is also antiviral and antifungal. *Virgin* coconut oil means that the oil has been extracted by a method that does not involve high heat and harmful chemicals. *Most commercial coconut oil is refined, bleached, and deodorized, so read the label to make sure you are buying virgin coconut oil.*

Palm Kernel Oil

Palm oil, which is widely consumed in Africa and Asia, is extracted from the seed of the palm fruit, which is very oily. Some European food manufacturers are now using it in their baked food products and snack foods. Palm oil is also high in lauric acid.

Organic Cold-Pressed Sesame Oil

People have been consuming sesame oil for more than five thousand years. During the 1930s sesame oil was in wide use in the United States, and we were importing huge amounts of sesame seeds every year. After World War II the use of *inexpensive soybean and cottonseed oils* became prevalent. These oils are now genetically modified and should not be consumed. Sesame oil is trans-fat-free and contains sesamol and sesamin, natural antioxidants found in both the oil and the seeds. Sesame oil is an essential ingredient in Asian cooking and is adaptable to all kinds of cooking.

Ghee, Better than Butter

I use ghee in my cooking and love its wonderful buttery flavor. Ghee is also known as clarified butter. To make ghee, butter is slowly simmered in a saucepan over low heat until three layers form. The top layer is foamy and is skimmed off. The middle, liquid gold layer is the ghee. The bottom layer, the milk solids, sink to the bottom of the pan. Ghee will not burn while sautéing—it has a very high smoke point, and its chemical structure does not change at high heat. Because all the milk proteins have been removed during the clarifying process it is casein- and lactose-free. Ghee can be used in the same way as butter. Ghee, made from pastured butter, contains CLA and the fat-soluble vitamins A, D, E, and K_2 (activator X).

To make ghee, simply simmer 1 pound of pastured butter for about twenty minutes. Skim foam as necessary. When clarified, strain and store in small jars. Keep one jar near the stove for cooking (it does not need refrigeration) and the remaining jar in the refrigerator for future use.

Goose and Duck Fat

Duck and goose fat can usually be found at your local gourmet market. These rendered fats are delicious and can be used for sautéing. You can also render your own chicken fat for cooking if duck and goose fat are not available.

Pig's Lard

It's difficult to find pig's lard that comes from *pastured* pigs (humanely raised and without preservatives), therefore I have not included its use in the recipes in this book. For locally produced lard from pastured pigs you might try contacting your local chapter of the Weston A. Price Foundation. You can also check the classified ads in *Wise Traditions,* the foundation's quarterly magazine.

Seasonings and Condiments

Fresh herbs, spices, and appropriate dressings make all the difference in the flavor of a dish. Below are the most basic but important items to stock on your shelf.

Spices and Herbs

I recommend that your spices be organic. Peppercorns are one of the most heavily pesticide-sprayed crops. Freshness is also important for your spices. Freshly ground pepper makes all the difference in cooking. Get a good pepper grinder and keep it handy. If you have a small space outside your kitchen to grow fresh herbs, they will add wonderful flavors to your dressings and sauces. I keep ginger in the freezer, take it out as needed and grate it with a microplane grater then immediately return it to the freezer. The following are the spices and herbs I usually keep available.

- cinnamon
- coriander
- allspice
- ground cumin
- cardamom
- paprika
- fresh thyme
- ground ginger
- fresh cilantro

- nutmeg
- Tellecheri peppercorns
- bay leaves
- turmeric
- red chili flakes
- fresh oregano
- Madras curry powder
- ground cloves
- fresh basil

A Selection of Salts

It's fun to have a variety of salts on hand to flavor a dish. These are some basic ones that I use, but there are many interesting ones available now at most gourmet stores, so try some out.

Celtic sea salt comes from one of the most pristine coastal regions of France and is my most recommended sea salt. It is harvested by a method that preserves its purity and balance of ocean minerals. Celtic sea salt contains higher levels of minerals and other trace elements than all the other sea salts. It is especially good with fish. Try the Flower of the Ocean finishing salt to add sparkle to salads and veggies.

Himalayan pink salt is hand mined. This 250-million-year-old, ancient sea salt is harvested from the foothills of the Himalayas and is unrefined and unpolluted. It is one of the purest salts in the world and is reported to contain eighty-four trace elements.

Redmond sea salt—from a small town near Redmond, Utah—is an unrefined pure sea salt from an ancient inland seabed. This beautiful pink salt is extracted from deep within the earth. It is not bleached, kiln dried, heated, or altered with pollutants. Redmond salt also has a full complement of trace minerals. It is relatively inexpensive. I always have it next to the stove in a little dish for daily cooking.

A Variety of Vinegars

I love to flavor my homemade dressings with interesting vinegars. Acidity is what makes a vinegar stand out. A great vinegar imparts fruitiness, fragrance, and depth to a dish. There are many varieties to choose from, such as seasoned organic brown rice wine vinegar, organic apple cider vinegar, aged balsamic vinegar, red wine vinegar, Spanish sherry vinegar, and Champagne vinegar. For more interest you might want to try American Balsamic from New Mexico, Traditional Aceto Balsamico of Monticello, Datu Puti Coconut Vinegar from the Philippines, Gold Plum Chinkiang Vinegar from China, or an unfiltered, unpasteurized apple cider vinegar from Quebec such as Verger Pierre Gingras Natural Handcrafted Cider Vinegar. I often use Bragg's Raw Unfiltered Organic Apple Cider Vinegar and Coconut Secret Raw Coconut Vinegar.

Sugar Substitutes

I recommend 100 percent pure stevia, with no fillers or other harmful ingredients, as an alternative sweetener. Stevia is a non-carbohydrate, non-caloric sweetener that can be used by those who cannot tolerate sugar or other sweeteners. I recommended using stevia "to taste" in many of the recipes that call for a sweetener. A recommended organic brand, Stevita (100% pure) also comes in flavors like Chocolate, Cognac, Mango, Orange, Peach, Peppermint, Strawberry, and Toffee. Stevita stevia is cultivated in one of the best and richest soils in the world (the southern Brazilian red clay soil) by Steviafarma, a company that is conscientious about the preservation of the environment and continuously searching for social harmony through spiritual, ecological, and sustainable industrial farming practices.

Chocolate

Everyone loves chocolate, and fortunately it is full of antioxidants and health-giving properties. Historically, chocolate has been known as "the food of the gods." When using chocolate in your cooking, I urge you to buy only organic cacao powder, chocolate bars, or nibs. There are several good brands on the market such as Z Natural Raw Organic Cacao Powder, Navitas Naturals Raw Power Organic Cacao Powder, Dagoba, Green and Blacks, and Holy Kakao Raw Organic Cacao Powder. *Organic* means that the workers (and their children) who harvest the cacao are not exposed to deadly pesticides. *Please pay attention to this.* Just because the label says Fair Trade does not mean it is organic. For more information go to www.transfairusa.org.

Say Cheese!

When I catered in the Napa Valley it was quite the norm to serve a cheese course, so I became familiar with many fine California and European cheeses. Dean & Delucca in St. Helena had an abundant cheese counter that I would swoon over. There was also a cheese man at the farmers' market who had a great selection of cheeses. He would admonish us *never* to wrap the cheese in plastic. In Europe the cheeses just sit out at room temperature.

Though California is now a major producer of artisanal and raw milk cheeses, many other states also produce raw milk cheeses. You can find raw milk cheeses at Trader Joe's, Whole Foods, Briar Patch Co-Op, Costco, and many local cheese shops. If you are a cheese lover it might be fun for you to go to your favorite cheese shop and do some tasting. The Resources section (page 260) also includes a comprehensive list of producers of wonderful raw milk cheeses. When you entertain, a fabulous selection of cheeses, unusual olives, and nuts will surely please your guests. I would rather have fine cheeses than most hors d'oeuvres any day. Please visit the Real Milk website or refer to the Resources section (page 260) for a list of raw cheese producers.

Nondairy Milks and Ice Cream

Nut milks and coconut milk are good substitutes for those who cannot have dairy. You can make your own nut milks by soaking the nuts overnight in filtered water. Puree the nuts in a blender with additional water and then strain the nut milk through a nut milk bag or a cheesecloth-lined sieve. It is better to make your own nut milks as many of the commercial nut milks are sweetened with cane juice and have high sugar content. I've also noticed that many of them are fortified with synthetic vitamins, which are best avoided. I've included a recipe for making almond milk in the breakfast section; you will find it is more flavorful and much creamier than store bought. Make sure the nuts you use are very fresh.

I'm happy to report that ice cream made with coconut milk is a spectacular alternative to conventional ice cream; it beats, hands down, soy ice creams and rice ice creams, which taste disappointing to say the least. I have included recipes in the dessert section for coconut milk ice creams. Sources for raw organic powdered coconut milk and coconut cream are Wilderness Family Naturals and Z Natural Foods. The taste of powdered raw coconut milk is so superior you will never go back to using canned coconut milk again. To make the milk just follow the easy package directions.

Raw Nuts and Seeds

Nuts and seeds are an excellent source of additional protein and essential fatty acids in the diet. Keep your pantry well stocked with fresh seeds such as sunflower, pumpkin, chia, sesame, and flax. Nuts would include "raw" organic almonds, walnuts, pine nuts, pecans, hazelnuts, and brazil nuts.

"Truly Raw" Almonds

It is highly unlikely if you are buying almonds labeled "raw" in California that they are *really raw*. From a whole, living-food perspective, the almonds are mislabeled. Unfortunately the USDA and the California Almond Board have approved this false labeling. Be warned that pasteurized almonds sold as raw have the potential to be toxic.*

Fortunately you can find safe and truly raw almonds on the market: D&S Ranch in California has developed a steam method to remove bacteria from their almonds. This method allows them to sell their almonds as truly raw, preserving the internal balance of enzymes, amino acids, and proteins. Because the almonds are not pasteurized you can actually sprout them.

For a selection of bulk organic almonds, pistachios, and walnuts please visit the Braga Organic Farms website, provided in the Resources section (page 258). For organic hazelnuts, I located Freddy Guys hazelnuts at the Portland Farmers' Market. Golden Omega Flax Seed is pesticide-free and can be purchased from Heavenly Harvest, Corvalis, Oregon.

---

*To read the whole story about the McAfee Farms and Organic Pastures Dairy position on the pasteurization of almonds go to http://organicpastures.com/raw_almonds.html.

Preparing Nuts and Seeds

Soaking the seeds and nuts in lightly salted water is an important step and will eliminate phytic acid and trypsin inhibitors. This is not necessary for Brazil nuts and hazelnuts, as they contain no enzyme inhibitors. Soaking begins the sprouting process so that all the important nutrition is made available.

SUGGESTED SOAKING TIMES

NUT/SEED	HOURS
Almonds	4–6
Cashews	4–6
Flax seeds	6
Pecans	2
Pumpkin seeds	4
Sunflower seeds	4
Walnuts	2

Rinse the seeds and nuts well after soaking, then dry on a sheet pan in a dehydrator, if you have one, or a 150 degree oven.

Olives

Artisanal cured olives are the perfect party food and can be an amazing conversation starter. If you want to learn about how wonderful all the varieties are, just go to the Whole Foods olive bar. You will be amazed at the selection. Some of my favorites are Manzanilla and Arbequina from Spain; Cerignola from Italy; and Picholine, Green Lucques, Niçoise, and black oil–cured from France. California will soon catch up on the gourmet table olives, too. Look for McEvoy Tuscan Table Olives and La Bella Gourmet California-grown olives.

Additional Paleo Pantry Items

I also suggest having the following items on hand.

- Pure organic extracts and flavorings
- Nutritional yeast

- Pomegranate molasses (middle Eastern stores or Whole Foods)
- Dijon and a variety of favorite mustards
- Coconut Secret, 100% gluten-free, Raw Coconut Aminos (to replace tamari and soy sauce)
- Anchovies or anchovy paste
- Japanese wasabi paste
- Red Boat Fish Sauce
- Mae Ploy, Thai red and green chili paste
- Mongolian Fire Oil
- Estancia Lucia Chimichurri Traditional Argentinean Sauce (to replace Worcestershire sauce)
- Canned chipotle chilies (Mexican)
- Roasted red peppers, in jars (if you do not want to roast your own)
- Organic plum tomatoes and tomato paste
- Organic frozen berries
- New Medica, 100% gluten-free Power Greens (berry, chocolate, mint)

SHOPPING FOR HEALTH

The first thing to do before you go shopping is to get rid of the foods you will not be using any longer. You will be throwing away processed, packaged, junk foods (most snack items), and fast foods. Don't be afraid to be ruthless. *Reading labels is the key.* By eliminating the foods that are not on your paleo plan for health you will be making space in your refrigerator and your pantry for only healthy foods.

It's best to do your major shopping once a week when you have the time to pay attention. Make a master list of all the ingredients you normally use, including grassfed and pastured meats and dairy, wild-caught seafood, organic fruits, vegetables, nuts, and seeds, seasonings, and condiments. From the list of suggested items for your pantry you can select the ones that become your favorites. Keep your master list handy as a reminder and check things off during the week that you will need. This way you will have your list ready.

The Nearest Farmers' Market
One place you might want to begin shopping is your local farmers' market, which is a wonderful place to learn about selecting, preparing, and preserving the bounty of your region. This is the best way to get acquainted with growers of organic

fruits and vegetables in your area. There will also be local producers of grassfed meats, cheeses, and pastured poultry and eggs. Most farmers' markets near the coast have vendors for sustainably fished, line-caught fish as well as shellfish. To help you find a farmers' market in your area, a National Directory of Farmers' Markets' is published annually by the USDA.

A Saturday at the farmers' market makes a great educational weekend event for children. Let them have the fun of picking out food for the week and tasting some treats. This is a wonderful way we can teach our children where food comes from and what quality ingredients should be in our diet. They will also learn to recognize all the varieties of vegetables and fruits.

Neighborhood Grocery Stores

Fortunately we now have stores like Whole Foods, Trader Joe's, Briar Patch Co-Op, New Seasons, and Wild Oats, which carry most of the products that will make it easy for you to do your shopping. Even major stores, like Safeway and Costco, are joining the organic mainstream. Be active and tell your grocery store manager what you want. The main focus, other than reading labels, is to buy nonpackaged whole organic foods.

Buy Fresh, in Bulk, and Local

Every year we contribute mountains of metal, glass, paper, cardboard, and plastic to our growing landfills. Even if we recycle, this practice of packaging everything costs

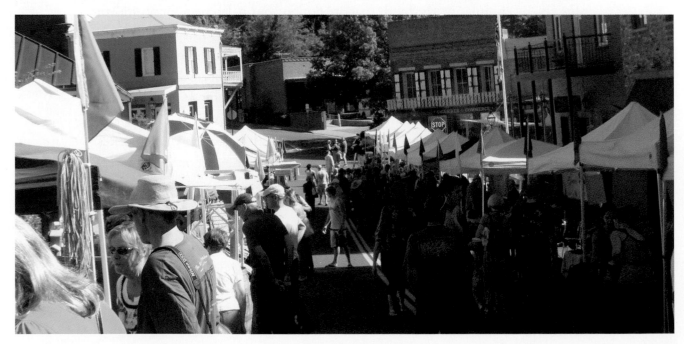

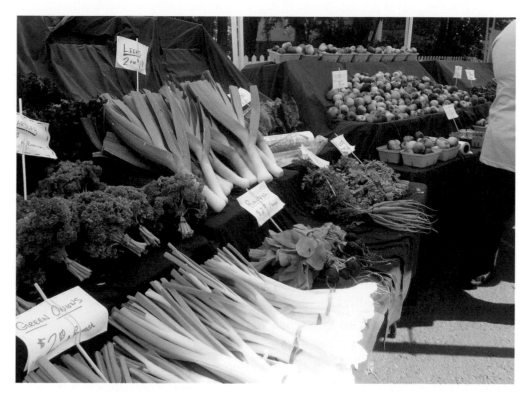

us in ways that we don't realize. The cost of the oil used to transport all this packaged food and then to transport the resulting garbage and recycling cannot be overlooked. This is a major reason to stop using prepackaged foods as much as possible.

You may want to form or join a food coop and buy in bulk or buy directly from the producers. This could add up to tremendous yearly savings on your food budget as well as saving the environment. One of the most inspiring books about eating locally grown food is *Animal, Vegetable, Miracle* by Barbara Kingsolver. Following her example of learning to live close to your food source—and enjoying it—is worth a try. Take a look at each product you use and try to choose items that at least come from the state in which you live.

Grow Your Own

Another wonderful option is to grow your own herbs and vegetables. Favorite herbs to grow would be sage, rosemary, marjoram, oregano, a variety of thyme, and various mints. If you live in a region where you can grow your own basil, grow as much as you can to make pesto to freeze for use during the year. You can never have enough basil.

Growing vegetables is a wonderful way to teach your children where their food comes from. There are so many varieties of heirloom seeds nowadays, so let the kids have the joy of selecting what they want to grow. If you live in a city there are now many urban gardens you can participate in. Also, saving your seeds or purchasing heirloom seeds from reputable seed companies is a way to ensure the viability of our future seed supply. Monsanto is very busy buying up seed supplies with the goal of patenting seeds for profit.

■ ■ ■

Before continuing on to the recipe section I would like to remind you that the protein content of the recipes has been reduced to remain within the guidelines of no more than 25 grams of pure protein per meal. So if you don't see the usual 6- to 8-ounce per person portions of meat or fish in a recipe, don't think I have made a mistake. Personally, I eat small protein snacks during the day to keep my blood sugar in balance. This way, when you sit down to lunch or dinner you are not starving and inclined to overeat at one sitting.

Also, I have been very careful with the recipes to make many substitution suggestions for those who have food sensitivities or allergies, especially when it comes to gluten or casein. Every product recommended in this book has been screened to be 100 percent gluten-free. Nora has been very kind to recommend some of her favorites. As for cheeses, you will know whether you can still incorporate dairy products in your diet. If you are having unexplained symptoms, please stay safe and get tested.

Enjoy the recipes and don't be afraid to experiment with your own flavor ideas. That's the fun of cooking.

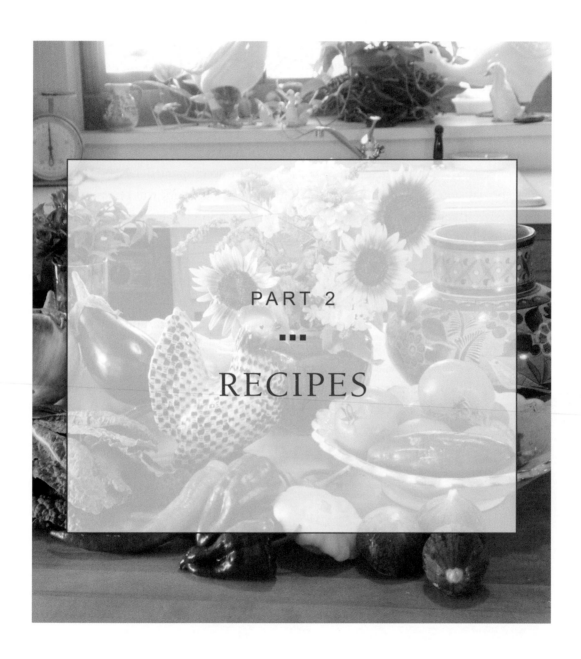

PART 2

• • •

RECIPES

A GOOD BREAKFAST

Everyone needs a high-energy breakfast of protein accompanied by good fats to start the day and carry you through until lunchtime. Your work will be much more productive if your brain has gotten the supporting nutrients it needs to function properly. Children especially need a good protein breakfast for their developing brains and to help them do well in school. Remember that what you eat affects mood and behavior during the day. If you begin the day with a high-protein smoothie or some meat and eggs, you will not only have better energy, you will be able stay sated longer and not be subject to cravings for unhealthy snacks later in the morning. Let's all have a good paleo breakfast to begin the day!

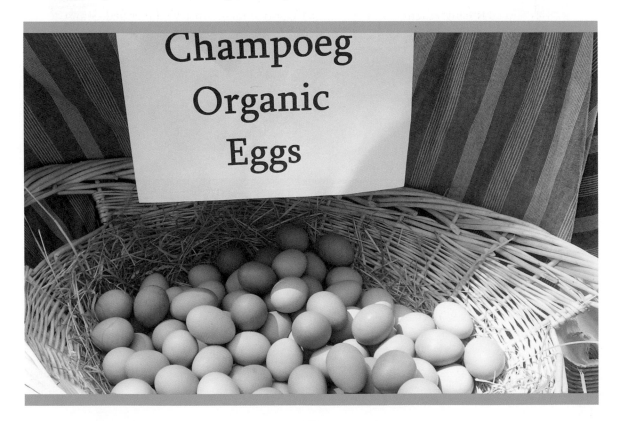

Homemade Almond or Hazelnut Milk

MAKES 1 QUART

You can buy organic, unsweetened almond milk, or you can make your own. Many store-bought nut milks, even though they are organic, contain high amounts of cane juice, rice starch, vegetable gums, and synthetic vitamins, so read labels carefully. You won't want to buy boxed almond milk at the store after you've made it yourself. Your smoothies will definitely taste better. Nut milks are a great alternative to cow's milk or cream. Use the nut milk for hot chocolate or in your ice cream recipes.

1 cup raw almonds or hazelnuts*

4 cups filtered water

2 tablespoons virgin coconut oil, melted

Stevita[†] stevia, to taste (optional)

½ teaspoon vanilla

pinch of sea salt

Soak the almonds 4 to 6 hours in lightly salted water to remove phytates and enzyme inhibitors. Rinse the nuts thoroughly before making the nut milk.

Blend all the ingredients in a blender or Vitamix on high until well blended. Strain the mixture through a nut milk bag or cheesecloth draped over a sieve. Use a spoon to press out as much of the milk as possible. Store the nut milk in a glass jar in the refrigerator until ready to use.

You can toast the leftover pulp on a sheetpan in the oven and use it for other recipes, such as Nora Gedgaudas's Coconut Bliss Truffles (page 247), a nut crust, or as a topping on yogurt or fruit. Freeze in zip-top bags until ready to use.

---

*Read about Truly Raw almonds on the Organic Pastures Raw Dairy website: www.organicpastures .com. Hazelnuts do not have to be soaked prior to making hazelnut milk, because they do not contain enzyme inhibitors.

[†]Stevita brand stevia is known to be organic and 100% pure stevia with no additives. It is the recommended brand for the recipes in this book. Stevita comes in delicious flavors that you may want to try for added interest in the recipes.

Dairy Cream Substitute—Coconut Milk

Coconut milk is a recommended cream substitute from Nora Gedgaudas: "I've taken to using pure coconut milk as a substitute for dairy cream, and I don't even miss the dairy cream. It's amazing. One can use either just the solid portion of canned coconut milk or the coconut cream made by Wilderness Family Naturals. I've also blended coconut milk with organic, unsweetened almond milk and alcohol-free vanilla extract for a bit of a cream or half-and-half substitute."

Coconut milk has a subtle coconut flavor and is slightly richer tasting than most other nut and seed milks, because of its high fat content. It can be used as a milk substitute in recipes, poured over cereal, or used as a beverage. It blends well in hot liquids and can also be used as a creamer in coffee. I use organic coconut milk powder, which can be purchased from Wilderness Family Naturals or Z Naturals. There are several brands on the market, so use your favorite. The package directions for making coconut milk are simple: just blend the coconut powder with warm water. I always have freshly mixed coconut milk in the fridge for ice creams, puddings, soups, and smoothies. You will never go back to canned coconut milk again.

Coconut Cream and Coconut Whipped Cream

Coconut cream is made the same way as coconut milk except that it has a higher fat content, giving it a richer, creamier texture. It is great used as a coffee creamer or poured over berries for dessert. You can even whip it for a whipped cream substitute, which is certainly healthier than some other whipped cream alternatives.

Coconut Whipped Cream
Serves approximately 8–10

Coconut whipped cream may be used as a replacement for dairy whipped cream.

> 1 carton (8 ounces) Wilderness Family Naturals
>   Coconut Cream
> Stevita stevia, to taste
> 1 teaspoon vanilla

Pour the carton of coconut cream into a chilled mixing bowl. Whip on high with an electric hand beater for 1 minute or so, until the cream begins to stiffen. Add the stevia and vanilla and beat again until soft peaks form.

Place the bowl in the refrigerator for 10–15 minutes and then beat again, until stiff peaks form, about 1 minute.

Komodo Dragon's Milk

For kids of all ages

SERVES 1

Did you know dragons make colorful milk? This morning drink has protein and important green nutrients. It's an easy way to get the kids to have their greens. Nu Medica, 100 percent gluten-free power greens, come in chocolate, mint, and berry flavors. Also, I invite you to learn about another wonder plant recommended in this recipe, Moringa oleifera, which is found in the optional moringa powder.*

> 1 teaspoon (or more) NuMedica 100 percent gluten-
> free Power Greens or 1 teaspoon organic moringa
> powder
> 1 cup almond milk, well chilled
> 1 tablespoon raw almond butter
> ½ cup favorite organic fresh or frozen berries (optional)
> Stevita stevia, to taste
> ½ teaspoon vanilla

In a blender blend together all ingredients. Add more almond milk if necessary.

---

*Moringa is an amazing plant. To learn about this highly nutritious plant go to www.organicmoringausa.com.

Chocolate Chai
SERVES 2 GENEROUSLY

This is a very unusual, fragrant, and spicy beverage for cold winter mornings and is great when curling up with a good book! In the summer you can chill the chai and serve it in frosty glasses. Choose the spices that please your taste buds.

1 black tea tea bag
½ cup boiling water
2 tablespoons organic unsweetened cocao powder
Stevita stevia, to taste
¼ teaspoon ground nutmeg
⅛ teaspoon ground pepper
¼ teaspoon cinnamon
1 to 2 teaspoons microplaned fresh ginger
2 cups organic almond milk
1 teaspoon vanilla

Drop the tea bag into boiling water and let it steep for 5 minutes. Remove the bag.

In a saucepan combine the cocao powder, stevia, and spices. Stir in a little of the hot tea and mix into a paste. Whisk in the almond milk and the steeped tea. Heat the mixture until very hot, being careful not to boil. Remove from heat and add the vanilla. Pour the chai into mugs and garnish with more freshly ground nutmeg if desired.

Caliente Mexican Chocolate
SERVES 2

Hot chocolate is no longer just a drink for the kids. Authentic Mexican chocolate, which came from the Aztecs, is not very sweet and is made with dark chocolate, vanilla, ground almonds, and a variety of spices such as pepper, cinnamon, nutmeg, and chilies. All these ingredients are added to hot milk and then frothed with a hand-carved wooden tool called a molino. *You can buy a molino at a Mexican specialty food shop.*

4 tablespoons organic unsweetened cocao powder
Stevita stevia, to taste

2 cups almond milk

dashes of your choice of spices, such as cinnamon,
   nutmeg, ancho chili powder, ground pepper

½ teaspoon vanilla

Garnish: freshly grated nutmeg

Mix together the cacao powder, spices, and stevia in a small saucepan. Add a little almond milk to make a paste. Add the remaining almond milk and heat the mixture to the boiling point, whisking often. Add the vanilla and pour the hot chocolate into 2 mugs. Grate some nutmeg on the hot chocolate. For added flair, serve with cinnamon sticks.

Mint Chocolate Smoothie

SERVES 2

Keep glasses in the freezer, ready for your frosty smoothies.

2 cups well-chilled almond milk or coconut milk
   (chill in freezer for ½ hour, or until slushy)

2 teaspoons NuMedica gluten-free Power Greens
   (chocolate flavor) or organic moringa powder

2 tablespoons organic cocoa powder, if using a
   nonchocolate power green

½ teaspoon vanilla

Stevita stevia, to taste

8 spearmint leaves or ½ teaspoon mint extract,
   to taste

With the blender on high, mix all the ingredients well. Pour into frosty glasses.

Cardamom Lassi

SERVES 2

Lassi is a classic Indian beverage.

2 cups Capretta Rich and Creamy Goat Yogurt,*
organic raw kefir (quephor)† or coconut milk
Stevita stevia, to taste
1 scant teaspoon ground cardamom

Blend all ingredients in a blender until combined. Pour the Lassi into frosty glasses or place in the freezer for about 30 minutes until very cold.

Strawberry Sunrise

SERVES 2

This breakfast beverage is as beautiful as it is delicious. I like the whole-milk goat yogurt, which gives it a strawberry cheesecake flavor. If you are casein intolerant, use coconut milk or almond milk.

1 cup frozen organic strawberries
¾ cup freshly squeezed red grapefruit juice
½ cup Capretta Rich and Creamy Goat Yogurt,
Organic Raw Quephor, or coconut milk

Place all ingredients in a blender and puree until very smooth. Add a little more juice or water if the mixture is too thick. Serve in frosty glasses.

---

*Capretta Rich and Creamy Goat Yogurt is pasteurized.
†Organic Pastures raw cow's milk Quephor-brand kefir. Read about organic raw kefir on the Organic Pastures Dairy website: www.organicpastures.com.

Berry Smoothie

SERVES 2 TO 3

*Berries are high in antioxidants. I can't think of a healthier and
more delicious way to begin the day.*

1 cup frozen organic strawberries, marionberries,
   blueberries, or raspberries
Stevita stevia, to taste (optional)
2 tablespoons organic almond butter
2 cups almond milk, Organic Pastures raw milk,
   Organic Raw Quephor, or coconut milk

Blend ingredients, adding water if necessary to achieve a smooth consistency. Serve
in frosty glasses.

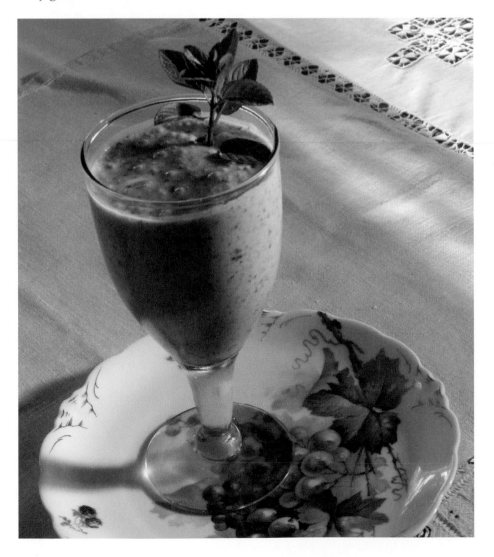

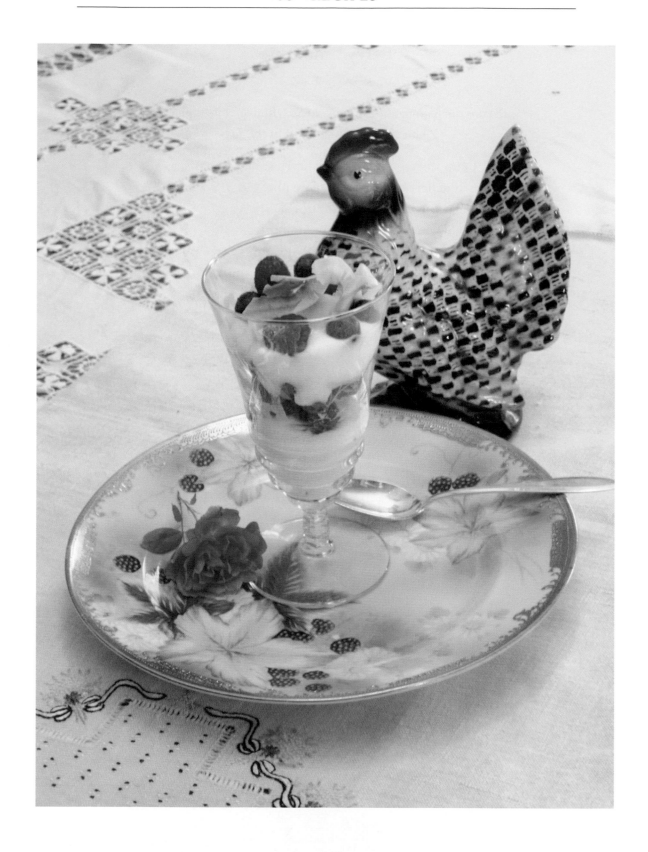

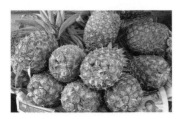

Frosty Piña Colada

SERVES 2

*Kids and grownups alike will love this
Piña Colada, served in tall frosty glasses
on a hot afternoon. Don't forget the umbrella.*

1 cup fresh or frozen organic pineapple chunks

8 ounces coconut milk

1 teaspoon vanilla

1 raw, pastured egg

Place the ingredients in a blender and puree until very smooth. With the blender running, add cold water until the mixture is the desired consistency.

Breakfast Fruit Compote

SERVES 2

Dessert for breakfast? Of course! This compote makes a nice brunch or luncheon dessert. The ripe fruit is sweet enough without additional sweeteners.

1 cup sliced organic strawberries, ripe summer
  peaches, or nectarines

¾ cup organic blueberries or raspberries

juice of ½ lime

½ cup Coconut Whipped Cream (see page 62) or
  Capretta Rich and Creamy Goat Yogurt

½ teaspoon vanilla extract

Garnish: toasted coconut, chopped almonds, dash of
  cinnamon, sprigs of mint for color

In a large bowl mix the fruit with the lime juice. In another bowl mix the whipped Coconut Cream or yogurt with the vanilla.

Using two glass tumblers or a widemouth wineglass and beginning with the fruit, layer the Coconut Whipped Cream or yogurt with the fruit. Garnish and serve with the sprigs of mint.

Scrambled Eggs with Caramelized Onions & Goat Cheese

SERVES 4

8 eggs, beaten

2 teaspoons fresh thyme

sea salt and freshly ground pepper, to taste

1 small, sweet onion, sliced

2 tablespoons ghee (see recipe for ghee on page 49)
    or cold-pressed sesame oil

4 ounces raw goat cheese crumbles or grated raw
    goat's milk cheddar*

In a bowl whisk together the eggs, thyme, salt and pepper. In a small skillet over medium heat, slowly sauté the onion in the ghee until very soft and caramelized. Remove the onions and set aside. In the same skillet add a little more ghee and cook the eggs until soft.

Divide the eggs onto plates and top with the caramelized onions and crumbled goat cheese or grated raw cheddar.

*Omit cheese if you are casein intolerant.

Egg and Vegetable Hash

SERVES 4

*Whatever vegetables you have left
from dinner can be thrown into this easy dish.*

2 tablespoons ghee or cold-pressed sesame oil

2 cups (approximately) leftover cooked vegetables

6 to 8 eggs, beaten

sea salt and freshly ground pepper, to taste

2 teaspoons minced parsley or other fresh herbs

Garnish: your favorite grated cheeses, Tabasco

Heat the oil in a heavy bottomed skillet, add the vegetables, and warm thoroughly. Increase the heat to medium. Pour the beaten eggs (seasoned with salt and pepper) into the skillet. Stir gently until they begin to set. Keep stirring the eggs until they are just done but still soft. Add the fresh herbs at the very end. Garnish with your favorite cheese. Serve immediately. Pass the Tabasco.

Poached Eggs with Asparagus
& Hollandaise Sauce

SERVES 4

Hollandaise sauce adds luxury to this simple breakfast. The goat's milk butter in this recipe is fabulous. You can also use wilted spinach or baby kale as the base for the eggs. This replicates eggs Florentine without the English muffin base. If you have leftover hollandaise, just refrigerate and use on your dinner veggies. For additional luxury, drape the asparagus with thin slices of prosciutto before placing the eggs on top.

8 pastured eggs, poached to desired doneness
1 bunch asparagus, ends trimmed and steamed
pinch of sea salt and a twist of pepper

Hollandaise Sauce

4 ounces pastured butter (Kerry Gold is a good
   brand) or Meyenberg Goat Butter
1 egg yolk
½ teaspoon Dijon mustard
2 tablespoons fresh lemon juice
pinch of sea salt
dash of cayenne or white pepper

In a small saucepan heat the butter to the boiling point. Place the egg yolk in the blender with the Dijon mustard and lemon juice. With the blender running slowly, pour in the hot butter until the hollandaise sauce emulsifies to the consistency of thin mayonnaise. You may not have to use all the butter. Season to taste with the salt and cayenne or white pepper.

To serve, divide the asparagus onto 4 plates. Top the asparagus with the poached eggs and a dollop of hollandaise sauce. Serve immediately, while hot.

Baked Eggs in Ramekins

SERVES 2

These eggs are wonderfully rich and creamy and will keep you satisfied for hours.

> 4 pastured eggs
> 4 tablespoons organic pastured cream
> pinch of sea salt and a twist of pepper
> Garnish: fresh chives, thyme, tarragon, savory, or
>   parsley, finely minced

Preheat the oven to 350 degrees. Liberally butter two 6-ounce ramekins. Place the eggs in the buttered ramekins. Place the ramekins in a baking dish half-filled with boiling water. Spoon the cream evenly over the tops of the eggs and sprinkle with salt and pepper. Bake the eggs for 15–20 minutes or until just set. Remove from the oven and sprinkle with the fresh herbs.

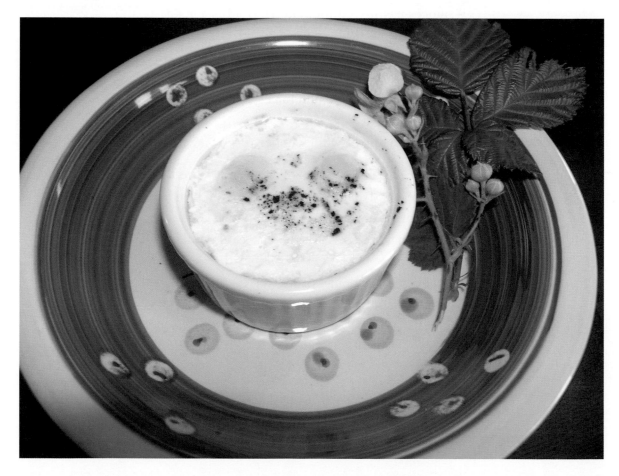

Japanese Scrambled Eggs

SERVES 4

Serve this Asian egg dish for an elegant Sunday brunch.

The Vegetables

2 to 3 tablespoons cold-pressed sesame oil

8 large shiitake mushrooms, sliced very thin

½ cup red bell pepper, sliced very thin

½ pound snow peas, sliced very thin on the diagonal

3 ounces pickled ginger, finely chopped

4 to 6 tablespoons Coconut Secret Raw Coconut
  Aminos, or to taste

2 tablespoons rice wine vinegar

The Eggs

8 eggs, beaten

2 teaspoons Coconut Secret Raw Coconut Aminos, or to taste

2 tablespoons sesame oil

Garnish: 2 scallions white and green parts, sliced
  very thin on the diagonal

For the vegetables: In a large sauté pan over medium heat, heat the sesame oil. Add the mushrooms and cook until soft. Add the bell pepper, snow peas, pickled ginger, coconut aminos, and rice wine vinegar. Mix well. Cover the pan and remove from heat. Keep veggies warm in pan.

For the eggs: In a bowl beat the eggs with the coconut aminos. In another sauté pan heat the sesame oil over medium heat, add the eggs, and scramble until just set.

To serve: Place equal portions of the warm vegetables on four plates. Top with the scrambled eggs. Garnish the eggs with the slivered scallions. Serve hot.

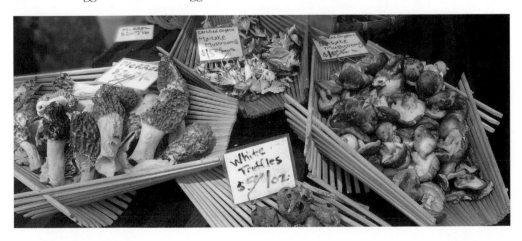

Fried Eggs with Asparagus
& Pecorino Romano

SERVES 2

This is a simple but elegant breakfast entrée that will surely impress. There are many varieties of sheep's milk pecorino romano. Duck eggs, if you can find them, are very rich compared to chicken eggs, so one per person will be enough. If you cannot have dairy try the Parmesan Cheese Substitute (page 152).

2 quarts lightly salted water

10 very fresh asparagus spears, tough bottom
   trimmed

6 tablespoons ghee, divided

pinch of sea salt and a twist of black pepper

4 pastured chicken eggs or 2 duck eggs

Garnish: grated sheep's milk pecorino romano or the
   Parmesan Cheese Substitute

In a medium saucepan bring the salted water to a boil. Blanch the asparagus for about 2 minutes or less, depending on the size of the spears. Remove the spears immediately and plunge them into ice water.

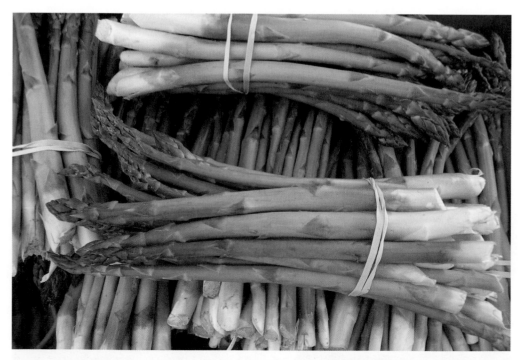

In a heavy-bottomed skillet on high heat, warm 3 tablespoons of ghee and heat the asparagus spears, coating them well. Season with the salt and pepper. Remove the spears and fan them out onto 2 dinner plates. Keep the plates in a warm oven while you cook the eggs.

After wiping out the skillet with a paper towel, add the remaining ghee and heat the pan to medium. Crack the eggs in the pan, taking care not to break the yolks. Cook the eggs gently, sunny side up, until the whites are done. Season the eggs with salt and pepper.

To serve, remove the eggs carefully with a wide spatula and place them on top of the asparagus. Grate the pecorino generously over the dish or use the Parmesan Cheese Substitute.

Huevos Mexicanos

SERVES 2

Protein to go! This is a great, hearty breakfast for teenagers on the move.
Serve with Caliente Mexican Chocolate.

    4 pastured eggs, beaten
    1 teaspoon pastured butter, ghee, or cold-pressed
        sesame oil
    pinch of sea salt and a twist of pepper
    Garnishes: your favorite grated cheese (try raw
        cheddar or jack, or crumbled goat cheese), finely
        chopped scallions, organic cherry tomatoes
        (halved), cilantro leaves, slices of avocado, or
        prepared guacamole

Prepare the bowls of garnishes.

In a skillet over medium heat melt the butter and cook the eggs until they reach the desired doneness. Salt and pepper to taste. Garnish with your choice of ingredients and a selection of favorite salsas. If you like your eggs over easy, this will work too.

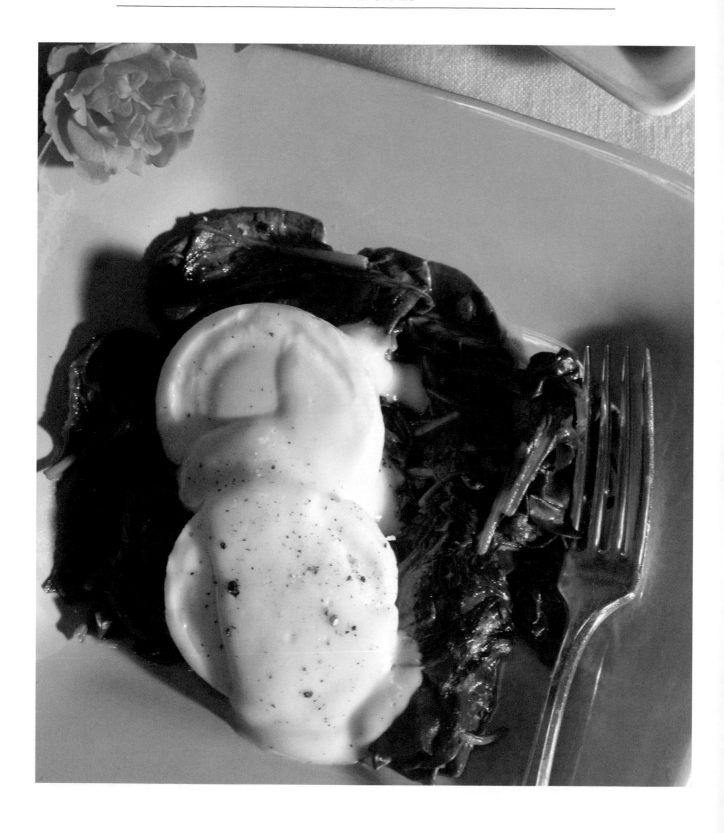

Poached Duck Eggs with Spinach & Pecorino Hollandaise

SERVES 4

*Fabulously rich! The sauce is also great on grilled or
steamed vegetables or fish!*

The Poached Duck Eggs with Spinach

1 heaping handful of baby spinach (per person)

4 tablespoons pastured butter or ghee

1 duck egg or two pastured chicken eggs (per person)

pinch of sea salt and a twist of pepper

Garnish: pecorino romano

The Pecorino Hollandaise Sauce

4 ounces pastured butter or Meyenberg Goat Butter

1 egg yolk

½ teaspoon Dijon mustard

2 tablespoons fresh lemon juice

3 tablespoons freshly grated sheep's milk pecorino romano

pinch of sea salt

dash of cayenne or white pepper

For the poached duck eggs: In a vegetable steamer over boiling water quickly wilt the spinach and remove to bowl. Keep warm.

In a large, heavy-bottomed skillet over medium-high heat melt the butter. Crack the eggs into the pan and cook them for 4–5 minutes without turning them (note that chicken eggs cook in less time) until the white is done. Season with salt and pepper.

For the pecorino hollandaise sauce: In a small saucepan heat the butter to boiling. In a blender place the egg yolk, Dijon mustard, lemon juice, and pecorino romano. With the blender running, slowly dribble in the hot butter until the hollandaise sauce emulsifies to the consistency of thin mayonnaise. You may not have to use all the butter. Season to taste with salt and pepper.

To serve: Place the spinach on 4 plates. Place the eggs on top of the spinach. Spoon a dollop of the pecorino hollandaise on each egg. Grate additional pecorino lavishly on top for garnish.

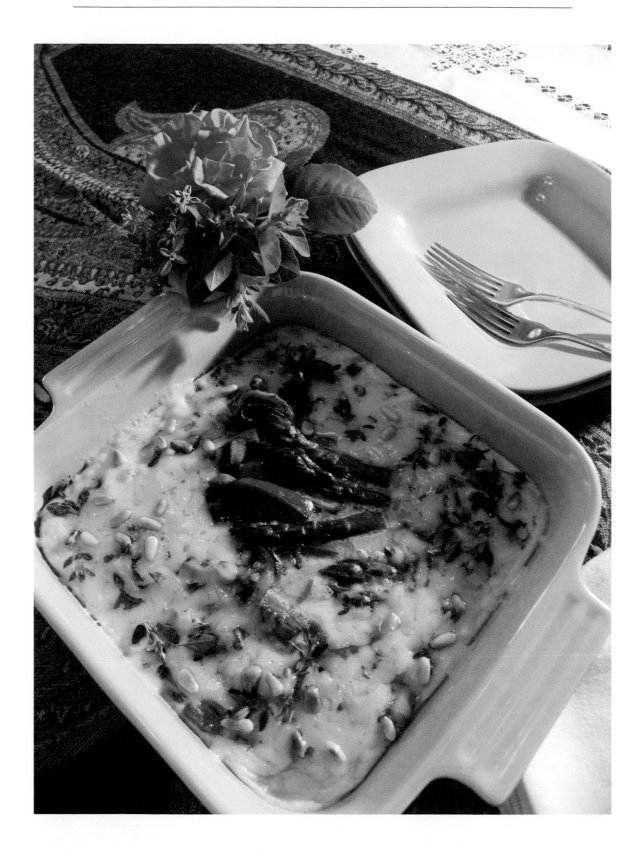

Vegetable Frittata

SERVES 4 TO 6

This is a great way to get vegetables into the kids. The nice thing about this frittata is you can use all your favorite vegetables.

The Eggs

    8 pastured eggs

    ½ teaspoon sea salt and a twist of pepper

The Vegetables

    ¼ cup pastured butter, ghee, or cold-pressed sesame
       oil

    ½ teaspoon sea salt

    4 cups cooked vegetables (sautéed onions, peppers,
       mushrooms, spinach or kale, broccolini, or
       asparagus)

The Topping

    ¼ cup favorite fresh herbs, such as parsley, basil,
       thyme, cilantro, or oregano, chopped

    ½ cup of grated cheese or Parmesan Cheese
       Substitute (page 152)

Preheat the oven to 325 degrees.

For the eggs: In a large bowl whisk together the eggs, salt, and freshly ground pepper. Set aside.

For the vegetables: In a 12-inch heavy bottomed stainless steel skillet heat the butter or ghee over medium-high heat. When the pan is hot add the onions, peppers, and mushrooms and cook about 15 minutes. Add the remaining ingredients and cook until the desired doneness.

For the frittata: Pour the whisked eggs into the skillet over the vegetable mixture. Bake the frittata, uncovered, about 15–20 minutes or until just set. Remove from oven and turn the oven to broil.

For the topping: Combine the topping herbs and the cheese in a bowl and evenly distribute the mixture over the top of the frittata. Place the skillet about 5 inches from the broiler and slightly brown the topping. Do not walk away while doing this step. Remove the frittata from the oven.

To serve: Cut the frittata into wedges and place on luncheon plates. Serve immediately. Pass more grated cheese if you like.

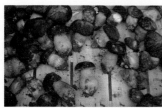

Wild Mushroom & Roasted Garlic Frittata

SERVES 4 AS AN ENTRÉE

This is an easy, festive, and flavorful
brunch dish. Serve the frittata with a
refreshing salad with the Citrus Vinaigrette (page 121).
Make the roasted garlic about an hour in advance
so it's ready for the remaining preparation.

The Roasted Garlic

1 head roasted garlic, about 10 cloves

1½ pounds crimini or shiitake mushrooms, thinly
   sliced

¼ cup pastured butter or ghee

2 scallions, minced

¼ cup fresh basil, julienned

The Eggs

8 pastured eggs

½ teaspoon sea salt and a twist of pepper

The Frittata Topping

2 jalapeño chilies, seeded and finely diced

¼ cup cilantro leaves, chopped

2 ounces crumbled goat cheese at room temperature

2 tablespoons toasted pine nuts or almonds, chopped

Preheat the oven to 325 degrees. Squeeze the roasted garlic out of the skin and mash. Set aside.

In a small bowl combine the minced scallion and the julienned basil. Set aside.

In a small bowl mix the diced jalapeños, chopped cilantro, crumbled goat cheese, and pine nuts. Set aside

In a large bowl whisk the eggs with the salt and pepper. Set aside.

In a 12-inch heavy bottomed stainless steel skillet heat the butter or ghee over medium-high heat. When hot add the mushrooms and roasted garlic and cook until very soft, about 15 minutes.

Sprinkle the scallions and julienned basil on top of the mushroom-garlic mixture and then pour the whisked eggs over the top. Bake the frittata in the preheated oven, uncovered, about 15 minutes or until just set. Remove from the oven and turn the oven on to broil.

Evenly distribute the topping mixture over the top of the frittata. Place the skillet about 5 inches from the broiler and cook long enough to melt and slightly brown the goat cheese. Watch this step carefully. Remove the frittata from the oven.

To serve, cut the frittata into wedges and place on 4 luncheon plates. Serve immediately.

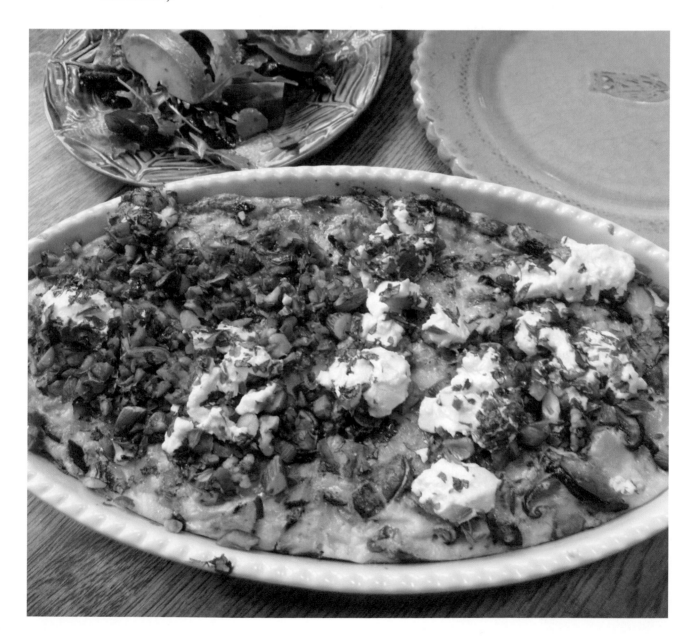

The Breakfast Bar

Here's a great way to stay organized for a family on the go: Have a large tray that sits on the counter. On the tray place glass jars filled with seeds and nuts so your family can use anything they want on their morning yogurt, in their smoothies, or on their salads at lunch.

Favorite tray items
pumpkin seeds

sunflower seeds

pecans

walnuts

raw almonds

pine nuts

organic dried coconut flakes.

I also grind chia, sesame, and flax seeds together and keep them in a jar in the refrigerator to add to the tray.

Have on hand in the refrigerator
coconut milk and coconut cream

raw milk

organic pastured cream

butter

almond milk

berries

pastured eggs

leftover veggies

organic almond butter

a jar of Parmesan Cheese Substitute (see page 152)

Once everything is on the counter, everyone can easily choose his or her own favorite paleo breakfast items.

Make it one of the kids' daily jobs to keep the jars filled from the main stock in the pantry. I haven't included dried fruit to the tray list because it has added sugars (28 grams per ounce). Better to use fresh or frozen berries.

PALEO PARTY

When I had my catering company, The Best of Everything, in the Napa Valley, I was known for my innovative hors d'oeuvres and dips, some of which I marketed in the local grocery stores. I've made all the recipes in this section Paleo "kosher." For crackers, I recommend Lydia's Organics Sunflower Seed Bread or Livin' Spoonful Sprouted Crackers. You can purchase the cookbook *Everyday Raw* by Matthew Kenney and try making your own crackers and chips from the recipes in the book. Making your own crackers is a fun family project.

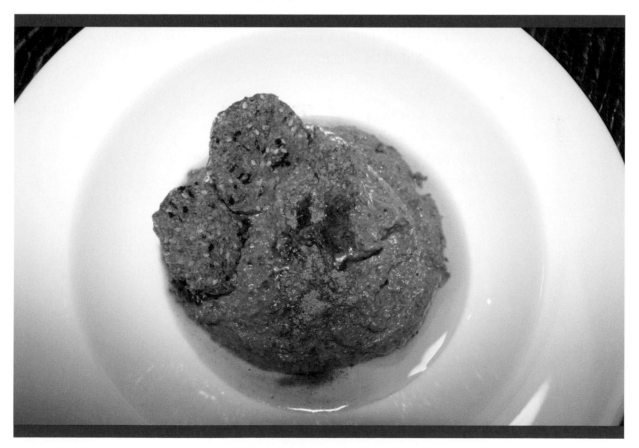

Party Nut Mix

SERVES 6 TO 8

These nuts are great to keep around the house or to take to work for snacks.
To make them, follow the directions for soaking and drying the nuts.

⅛ teaspoon cumin (or more if desired)

⅛ teaspoon cayenne (or more if desired)

¼ cup coconut oil

1¼ cups *total* (¼ cup each raw cashews, almonds,
     pecans, walnuts, or pistachios)

Celtic Flower of the Ocean sea salt* or Maldon sea
     salt, to taste

Preheat the oven to 375 degrees.

In a saucepan warm the coconut oil and the spices. Place the nuts in a large bowl and pour the spiced oil over the nuts. Mix thoroughly to coat. Place the nuts on a stainless steel sheet pan and roast them in the oven until they're golden brown. Keep turning the nuts with a spatula while they roast. Remove the sheet pan from the oven and sprinkle the nuts with the Flower of the Ocean salt or Maldon salt.

---

*Celtic Flower of the Ocean and Maldon salt are finishing salts that resemble snowflakes. They add sparkle to any dish.

Roasted Garlic

SERVES 6

Roasted garlic is so simple to make, and your family and friends will love you for it. Spread roasted garlic on Lydia's Organics Sunflower Seed Bread or Livin' Spoonful Sprouted Crackers. You can also squeeze the garlic onto cooked vegetables. Use the leftover roasted garlic skins for your homemade chicken or vegetable stock.

6 large heads of garlic
¼ cup cold-pressed sesame oil
pinches of sea salt and twists of pepper for each bulb

Preheat the oven to 350 degrees. With a sharp paring knife cut the tips off each garlic section. Brush the heads liberally with the sesame oil. Sprinkle each head with salt and pepper.

Place the heads of garlic in a glass pie pan and cover them with aluminum foil. Bake them for 1–1½ hours until very soft. When the garlic is done, reserve the oil. Drizzle the oil over vegetables or use it when you make homemade mayonnaise.

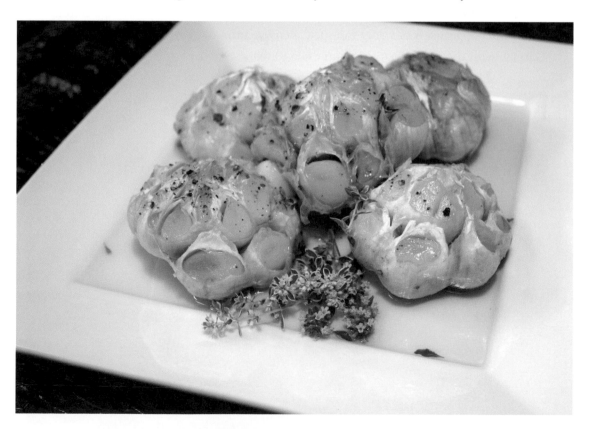

Toasted Goat Cheese

SERVES 6

This is a classic! Warm, toasted goat cheese is one of the joys of life. Serve the cheese with Lydia's Organics Sunflower Seed Bread or Livin' Spoonful Sprouted Crackers. Toasted goat cheese is the perfect accompaniment to a simple green salad.

½ cup toasted pecans, almonds, or macadamia nuts,
   ground in a food processor
3 tablespoons cold-pressed sesame oil
6 ounces soft goat cheese log, sliced into 6 rounds
Garnish: roasted garlic or oil-packed sun-dried
   tomatoes, sliced very thin

Preheat the oven to 400 degrees. Place the toasted ground nuts on a plate. Pour the sesame oil onto another plate. First, dip the cheese rounds in the oil and then the ground nuts. Place the rounds in a glass pie pan. You can refrigerate the cheese until ready for baking.

In the preheated oven toast the cheese rounds for 3–4 minutes, watching carefully so the cheese gets soft but does not melt. Remove from oven and serve immediately. Garnish with the roasted garlic or sun-dried tomatoes.

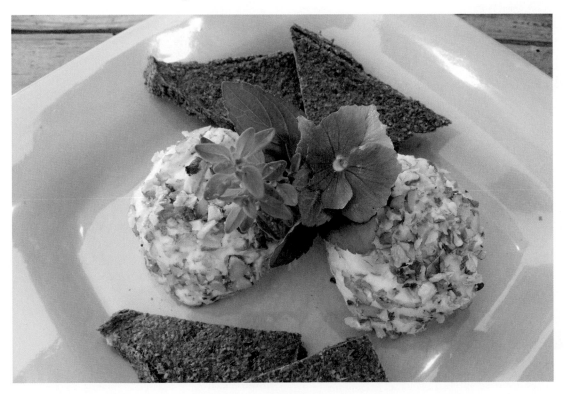

Bagna Cauda
(Italian Hot Olive Oil Sauce)

SERVES 4

The first time I ever tasted this sauce, I was about twelve years old. I was invited to my friend's house for dinner, and her mother served it. I couldn't stop eating. The recipe is from Piedmont, Italy, and translates as "hot bath." Serve the Bagna Cauda with plenty of raw or cooked vegetables as a party appetizer or serve it with your vegetables for dinner. Try it as a dipping sauce for steamed artichokes.

½ cup extra-virgin olive oil

4 ounces pastured butter or Meyenberg Goat Butter

6 cloves garlic, minced

⅛ teaspoon red chili flakes, optional

4 mashed anchovy fillets or 3 to 4 tablespoons
   anchovy paste (sold in a tube)

In a small saucepan over low heat warm the olive oil, butter, and garlic. Do not brown the garlic. Add the mashed anchovies or anchovy paste and the red chili flakes. Heat the mixture thoroughly. Transfer the bagna cauda to a heated bowl or fondue pot to stay warm.

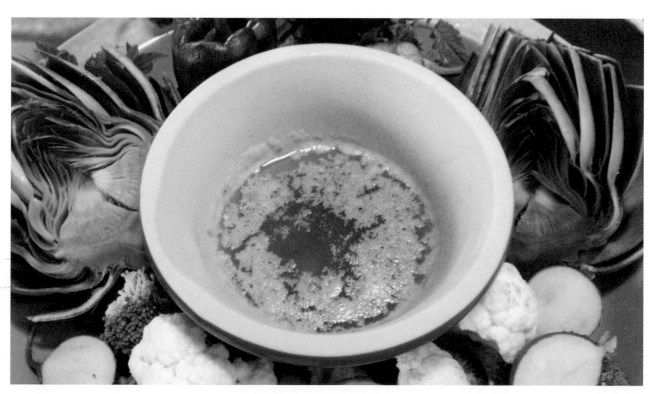

Coriander Marinated Olives

SERVES 8 TO 10

This recipe is very unusual. I use it to accompany the Mediterranean Spinach and Feta Salad (page 147). Marinate the olives for at least 8 hours so the flavors meld. You can find an extravagant olive selection at Whole Foods Market or at a specialty Italian deli.

½ pound cracked, but not pitted, Cypriot or
  cerignola olives
¼ cup extra-virgin olive oil
⅛ cup fresh lemon juice (use Meyer lemons, if
  possible)
3 to 4 cloves garlic, crushed
1 tablespoon whole cracked coriander seeds
½ lemon, cut into small wedges
1 fresh or dried bay leaf, cut into quarters

In a glass bowl combine all the ingredients. Cover and refrigerate for at least 8 hours, stirring occasionally. The olives will keep for a month. Bring them to room temperature before serving.

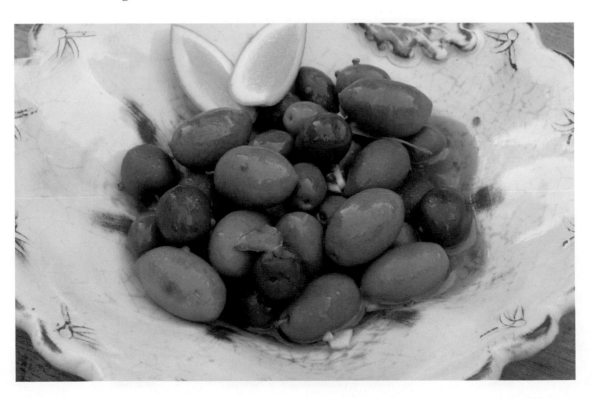

Olives with Orange and Fennel

SERVES APPROXIMATELY 10 TO 12

Olives make a healthy snack.
These olives are fragrant with fennel and orange.

4 organic oranges
2 medium fennel bulbs, cut lengthwise into eighths
¼ cup cold-pressed sesame oil
8 large cloves garlic, peeled and thinly sliced
½ teaspoon fennel seed, coarsely cracked
¼ teaspoon red pepper flakes
8 ounces each, French Piccoline, Greek kalamata,
    black oil–cured, and Spanish arbequena olives, or
    your favorite olive selection
Celtic Flower of the Ocean salt or Maldon salt

Put a large pot of water onto the stove and warm to medium heat. With a vegetable peeler, remove 16 strips of orange peel, each 2 inches long. Remove any white pith with a sharp paring knife.

Bring the pot of water to a boil. Add the fennel slices and cook for 3 minutes. Drain the fennel in a colander in the sink.

In a large saucepan over medium-high heat, warm the sesame oil. Add the orange peel, fennel slices, fennel seed, and red pepper flakes and cook until the mixture is sizzling, about 1 minute. Turn the heat down, add the olives and warm for about 5 minutes. Remove from heat and let the olives stand for about 6 hours, then discard the orange peel.

You can make the olives the day before the party. When you serve the olives, sprinkle lightly with your finishing salt. You can also use olives as a garnish with a green salad.

Magical Muhamara

SERVES 8 TO 10

I call this recipe, which originated in Syria, the "thinking man's" hummus.
It's my favorite dip. I packaged it and sold it under my The Best of Everything label in
the Napa and Sonoma areas. Serve the dip with special seeded crackers
or raw or cooked vegetables. It makes an unusual and delicious sauce for grilled fish.
For authentic flavor, you must use pomegranate molasses,
which is imported from the Middle East.*

1½ cups lightly toasted walnuts
4 large red bell peppers, roasted, skinned, and
   seeded (you can use roasted peppers in a jar)
2 teaspoons ground cumin
4 cloves garlic, minced
4 tablespoons pomegranate molasses
juice of ½ lemon
1 to 2 teaspoons red pepper flakes
¼ cup (or more) extra-virgin olive oil
sea salt and a twist of black pepper, to taste
Garnish: olive oil, ground cumin

Preheat the oven to 350 degrees. Place the walnuts on a sheet pan and toast in the oven for about 10 minutes, turning a few times so they toast evenly.

Combine all the ingredients, except the olive oil in a food processor. With the motor running, slowly pour in the olive oil and puree the mixture until very smooth. Adjust the seasonings to suit your taste. You may want more lemon, cumin, or garlic.

When serving, place the Muhamara in a bowl and drizzle a little olive oil over the top. Sprinkle some ground cumin on top for garnish.

Muhamara will keep in the refrigerator in a jar topped with olive oil for about two weeks. You can also freeze it.

---

*Pomegranate molasses is available at Whole Foods Market, Middle Eastern specialty food shops, and at www.chefshop.com.

Endive "Spoons" with Lemon Herb Goat Cheese

MAKES APPROXIMATELY 50 TO 60 "SPOONS"

This appetizer is simple to make but impressive to serve at a party. You can also serve the herbed cheese on cucumber slices.

1 pound goat cheese
2 tablespoons lemon juice
2 teaspoons lemon zest
2 tablespoons extra-virgin olive oil
3 tablespoons fresh chives, finely chopped
8 heads red or white Belgian endive
Garnish: 6 organic cherry tomatoes, sliced very thin,
    cilantro, or Italian (flat leaf) parsley (leaves only)

Blend goat cheese, lemon juice, lemon zest, and olive oil in a food processor. Stir in the chives. This can be done a day ahead of the party and refrigerated.

Before serving, separate the endive leaves and arrange on a platter. Place small amounts of the cheese mixture on the "spoon" end of the endive. Garnish each spoon with a slice of the tomato and a cilantro leaf.

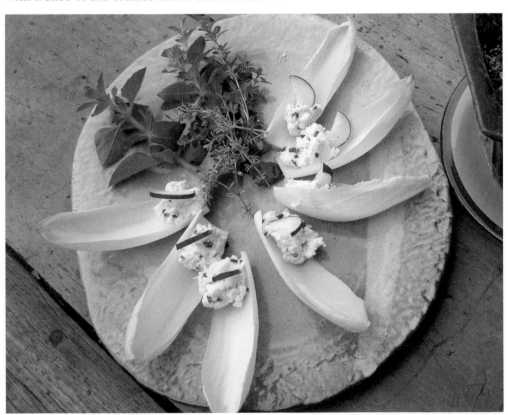

Pacific Rim Tuna Salsa

SERVES 8

This Asian tuna recipe will wake up your taste buds. It has sensational flavor, so make plenty. Serve it on cucumber slices or Lydia's Organics Sunflower Seed Bread. Tuna salsa may also be served on red leaf butter lettuce as a first course.

16 ounces sashimi-grade tuna (2 ounces per person if
    serving as an hors d'oeuvre)
1 ripe avocado, finely diced
juice of 4 to 5 limes
1 to 2 jalapeños, seeded and finely diced
3 tablespoons sesame oil
4 tablespoons raw cream or coconut milk
2 tablespoons sesame seeds
2 teaspoons Coconut Secret Raw Coconut Aminos,*
    or to taste
1 tablespoon grated fresh ginger, or to taste
8 heads red or white Belgian endive

Finely dice the tuna and place in a bowl. Add the remaining ingredients, except the endive. Stir very gently so you don't mash the avocado. You will want to see the avocado pieces clearly in the finished salad. Spoon this mixture onto the separated leaves of the endive. Sprinkle it with additional sesame seeds if desired. Serve immediately.

---

*Coconut aminos replace tamari for those who cannot consume foods containing gluten or soy.

Vegetable Platter with French Onion Dip

SERVES 6

Onion dip is always a party favorite. This dip is a great way to get the kids to eat their raw vegetables at dinner. Just make the dip and put their favorite vegetables on a platter. You can also serve the dip with Lydia's Organics Sunflower Seed Bread or Livin' Spoonful Sprouted Crackers.

The Vegetables

carrot and celery sticks, radishes, endive leaves, cauliflower florets, broccolini, or other vegetables of your choice

The Onion Dip

3 tablespoons cold-pressed sesame oil

2 medium onions, finely diced

5 ounces goat cheese, at room temperature

¾ cup raw cream or Homemade Mayonnaise (page 123)

¼ cup finely chopped chives

2 tablespoons fresh thyme leaves, chopped

2 tablespoons Champagne vinegar or white wine vinegar

sea salt and freshly ground pepper, to taste

In a sauté pan, heat the sesame oil and cook the onions slowly until caramelized and soft, approximately 30 minutes. Note: stir the onions so that they cook evenly. It's important to cook the onions slowly so the sugars release slowly and they maintain their sweetness. Remove them from heat and cool.

In a bowl mix the onions with the room temperature goat cheese and the cream. Add the herbs, vinegar, salt, and pepper. It's best to make the dip in the morning to give the flavors time to develop. Put the dip in a container with a lid and refrigerate until ready to serve.

Goat Cheese and Basil Dip

MAKES 2 CUPS

*This is a wonderful dip for party vegetables, but it is also great on
steamed asparagus or broccolini for dinner.*

½ cup Homemade Mayonnaise (page 123)
1 cup goat cheese, softened to room temperature
1 cup fresh basil leaves
½ cup raw cream
juice of ½ lemon
¼ teaspoon sea salt and a twist of pepper

Place all the ingredients in a food processor and blend until smooth.

Smoked Trout Paté

SERVES 4 AS AN APPETIZER

*Serve this easy paté on Lydia's Organics Sunflower Seed Bread,
rounds of English cucumber, or Belgian endive leaves.*

4 ounces smoked trout
½ cup Homemade Mayonnaise (page 123)
2 tablespoons extra-virgin olive oil
juice of ½ lemon, about 2 tablespoons
1 tablespoon creamed horseradish
¼ teaspoon cayenne

Place all the ingredients in a food processor and blend until the mixture is smooth,
about 1 minute. Transfer the mixture to a covered container and refrigerate it until
ready to serve.

Smoked Salmon with Spicy Mango Salsa

SERVES 8

This is a pretty and tastier version of the familiar smoked salmon and cream cheese. Serve it with Lydia's Organics Sunflower Seed Bread, Belgian endive leaves, or round slices of English cucumber. This appetizer can be served for lunch with a salad of lightly dressed greens. The goat cream cheese is very mild and tastes like a tangy cream cheese. If you can't have dairy, then omit the cheese. The salmon and the salsa are wonderful on their own.

The Salmon

10 ounces sliced smoked salmon

The Spicy Mango Salsa

2 mangoes, peeled, pit removed, and finely diced

2 scallions, white and light green part, minced

½ cup cilantro leaves, chopped

3 tablespoons fresh lime juice (1 large lime)

1 teaspoon Asian chili sauce

Garnish: additional cilantro leaves

The Goat Cream Cheese

8 ounces goat cheese, softened

3 to 4 tablespoons raw cream

In a bowl mix all the ingredients for the salsa and refrigerate until ready for use. In another small bowl beat the goat cheese and cream until light and fluffy.

To assemble the appetizer, spread some of the cream cheese mixture on the seed bread, a leaf of endive, or a round of cucumber and then lay a small piece of smoked salmon on top. Spoon a little of the mango salsa on top of the cilantro and garnish with a cilantro leaf.

Salmon Rillettes

MAKES 4 CUPS

Rillettes are a very rich and unusual French appetizer. Serve them with slices of English cucumber. It's best to prepare the rillettes the day before serving to let the flavors develop.

14 ounces canned wild Alaskan salmon

8 tablespoons pastured butter or Meyenberg goat butter, softened

½ cup raw cream or 4 ounces Meyenberg Crème de Chevre

2 tablespoons dry white vermouth

2 tablespoons fresh lemon juice

½ pound thinly sliced smoked salmon, finely diced

2 tablespoons capers, rinsed

1 bunch scallions, white and green parts, minced

½ cup fresh dill

pinch of cayenne and a twist of pepper

Garnish: 3 to 4 English cucumbers sliced on the diagonal about ¼-inch thick. Makes about 4 to 5 appetizers per guest.

In a food processor, puree the canned salmon, butter, cream, vermouth, and lemon juice until smooth. Remove the mixture to a bowl and fold in the diced smoked salmon, capers, scallions, dill, cayenne, and pepper. Mix until well blended. Taste the mixture for pepper balance. Pack the rillettes in an attractive crock or bowl, cover, and refrigerate.

To serve, let the rillettes come to room temperature. Place the crock or bowl on a large platter and surround it with the cucumber slices.

Grilled Prawns
Wrapped in Prosciutto

MAKES 2 TO 3 LARGE
PRAWNS PER PERSON

*Grilled prawns were always on my catering menu. They always
disappeared in a hurry. You can also wrap spears of asparagus with prosciutto.
Use the same method for grilling or broiling.*

prawns, raw
Italian Parma prosciutto slices
sesame oil
black pepper

Nothing could be easier. First, remove the tails from the raw prawns and devein them
with a sharp knife. Then cut the thinly sliced prosciutto into 1-inch-wide strips. Wrap
a strip around each raw prawn. Lay the prosciutto-wrapped prawns on a sheet pan
and brush them with sesame oil.

Grill or broil the prawns until done (when they lose their translucence). Turn
them at least once while grilling.

When they come off the grill, give them a couple twists of black pepper.

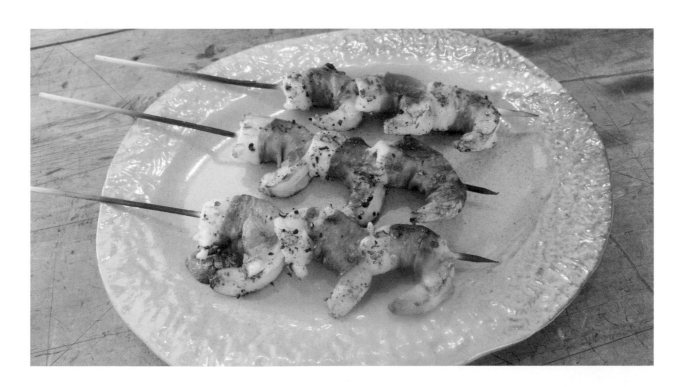

Thai Beef Satay

MAKES APPROXIMATELY 15

These delicious appetizers are served with Thai Spicy Almond Sauce (recipe below). They're a big hit at any party. You can serve them for dinner too. In this recipe the beef must marinate at least 2 hours or overnight.

The Meat and Marinade

1½ pounds of grassfed beef flank steak*

1¾ cups coconut milk

1 teaspoon Coconut Secret Raw Coconut Aminos

1 teaspoon yellow curry powder

1 teaspoon ground turmeric

1 teaspoon microplaned ginger

Garlic-Coconut Milk

½ teaspoon cold-pressed sesame oil

½ teaspoon minced garlic

¾ cup coconut milk

First, soak 15 long bamboo skewers in water for an hour.

In a bowl mix all the marinade ingredients. Then place the flank steak in a 9 × 13-inch glass baking dish and cover with the marinade. Marinate the steak in the refrigerator, covered, for about 4 hours, turning once to coat the meat thoroughly.

Mix together the garlic-coconut milk ingredients in a bowl. Set aside.

To prepare the skewers, cut the flank steak across the grain, holding the knife at an angle to the cutting surface so that each slice is about 1½-inches wide and ⅛-inch thick. There should be about fifteen or more strips. Thread each strip of beef lengthwise on a skewer. You may want to wrap the ends of the skewers in foil so they won't burn while grilling.

Start your grill on medium high. If you are using charcoal bring the coals to medium-high heat. Adjust the grill to about 4 inches above the coals. Place the skewers on the grill, as many as will fit.

While the satay skewers are cooking baste with the garlic-coconut milk. Grill the meat for about 1 minute until grill marks show and then turn and cook the other side for 1 minute, continuing to baste. Remove skewers from heat. Serve immediately with the Thai Spicy Almond Sauce (recipe follows).

---

*Chicken breast may also be used. After marinating, slice the breast across the grain as the above directions describe.

Thai Spicy Almond Sauce

MAKES APPROXIMATELY 4 CUPS

I used to go to a wonderful restaurant in Berkeley, Siam Cuisine, always with family or friends. All their dishes were first rate. We would order the grilled chili salad to see who could eat it without crying. It was always a tear jerker. Siam Cuisine had the best peanut curry sauce I've ever tasted, and this version, using almond butter, approximates the original. The almond sauce is also a great dip for raw vegetables. Because I have removed legumes from the recipes in this book and because some people are highly allergic to peanuts I have substituted almond butter for the usual peanut butter. I think it works very well.

¼ cup Mae Ploy Thai red curry paste (contains
   shrimp paste)
2 tablespoons Mongolian fire oil
1 tablespoon ground cayenne
1 tablespoon paprika (for color)
¾ teaspoon cinnamon
½ teaspoon ground cumin
⅛ teaspoon ground cloves
¼ cup Coconut Secret Raw Coconut Aminos, or to taste
5 cups coconut milk, divided
⅔ cup organic vegetable broth
2 tablespoons creamy almond butter

In a large saucepan combine the curry paste, Mongolian fire oil, cayenne, paprika, cinnamon, cumin, cloves, coconut aminos, and 1¾ cups of coconut milk. Bring the ingredients to a boil over medium heat and cook, stirring occasionally, for 5 minutes, until all the ingredients are well blended.

Add the vegetable broth and the remaining 3½ cups of coconut milk, 1 cup at a time, whisking with each addition. Continue cooking the sauce, while boiling gently, until it is reduced, about 25–30 minutes. Stir the sauce occasionally to prevent burning, adding more broth or water if necessary. At the end of the cooking time oil will appear on the top of the sauce. Just before removing from the heat, whisk the almond butter into the sauce until well blended.

To serve, pour the warm sauce onto a plate and dip the grilled beef or chicken satay in the sauce.

Scallop Ceviche with
Avocado-Mango Salsa & Belgian Endive

SERVES 8 AS AN HORS D'OEUVRE

I ate a lot of ceviche in Mexico. The local Mexicans would eat it for breakfast at a little
stand in La Penita de Jaltemba, where I had my house. The stand even served
a warm ceviche, which was quite unusual. This is a very colorful rendition
I know you will enjoy.

The Fusion Dressing
¼ fresh cilantro leaves, chopped

1 scallion, white and green parts, finely minced

1 clove garlic, minced

3 tablespoons fresh lime juice (1 large lime)

4 tablespoons cold-pressed sesame oil

1 teaspoon Asian chili sauce

1 tablespoon microplaned ginger

pinch of sea salt

The Scallop Ceviche and Avocado-Mango Salsa
16 ounces large day boat scallops, coarsely chopped

4 avocados, finely diced

1 red bell pepper, seeded and finely diced

2 ripe mangoes, peeled, pitted, and finely diced

juice of 2 limes

3 to 4 heads red or white Belgian endive leaves

Garnish: additional cilantro leaves

For the dressing: In a bowl whisk together all the dressing ingredients.

For the scallop ceviche and avocado-mango salsa: In a large bowl combine the scallops, avocados, red pepper, and mango. Squeeze the lime juice over the ingredients and mix gently. Pour the dressing over the scallops, mixing gently to not bruise the avocado and mango. Refrigerate the mixture until the hors d'oeuvres are ready to assemble.

To serve: Place a small amount of ceviche on each Belgian endive leaf and arrange the leaves on a colorful platter. Garnish each endive with a cilantro leaf.

SOULFUL SOUPS

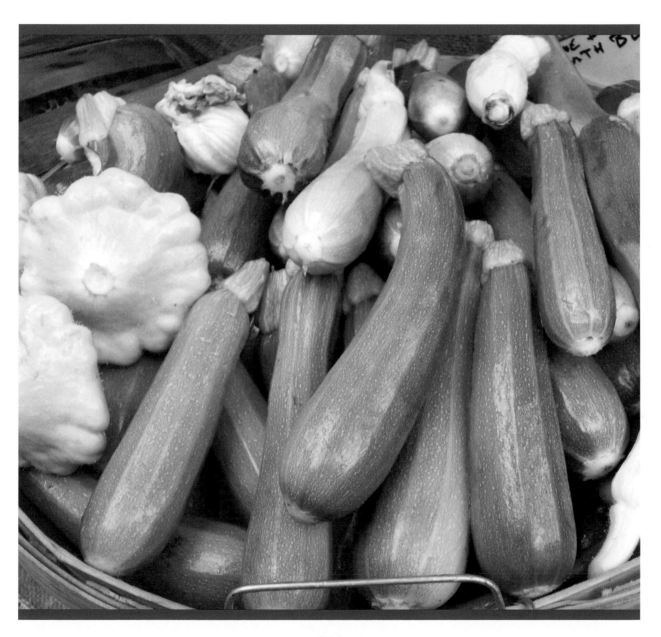

Homemade Stocks for Soup

I roast an organic chicken about once a week. The next day I make a rich chicken stock to have on hand for cooking vegetables and making soup. Sometimes I enjoy a cup of the stock by itself. Homemade stocks aid digestion and have been used for centuries as a remedy for illness and to soothe the digestive tract. Homemade stock is essential to flavor a good soup; it is full of vitamins and minerals and amino acids as well as other bioavailable nutrients. No wonder chicken soup is good for us when we're sick! Once you've made homemade stocks, you will never use store-bought broths again.

Chicken Stock

4 tablespoons cold-pressed sesame oil

4 cups sliced yellow onions or leeks, chopped*

2 cups carrots, chopped

2 cups celery and leaves, chopped

2 bulbs garlic, halved (also use leftover skins from
    Roasted Garlic (page 85)

5 to 6 pounds organic, free-range chicken bones,
    rinsed

2 large bay leaves

a few sprigs of fresh thyme

1 cup roughly chopped parsley

2 teaspoons sea salt

2 teaspoons whole black peppercorns

2 cups dry white wine, optional

1/4 cup raw apple cider vinegar

water to cover the ingredients in the pot by 3 inches,
    approximately 8 quarts

In a large stainless steel soup pot, lightly brown the vegetables in the oil. Add the chicken bones, herbs, seasonings, apple cider vinegar, and white wine. Cover the

---

*For an Asian version, replace the onions with scallions. Omit the bay leaves, parsley, thyme, and peppercorns. Instead, add three half-dollar-size slices of fresh ginger.

mixture with 3 inches of water, approximately 8 quarts. Bring the stock to a boil. Reduce heat and simmer, partially covered, for 4–6 hours. Skim the froth from the top of the stock as needed. Remove from heat when the stock is done. Cool and then strain through a large sieve into another pot. Using a measuring cup, portion the stock into glass Mason jars and use within a week or freeze for up to two months.

Hearty Vegetable Stock

¼ cup cold-pressed sesame oil

8 cups yellow onions, chopped (or a combination of onions and leeks)

4 cups carrots, roughly chopped

2 cups celery, tops and leaves, roughly chopped

1 cup each sliced celery root, fennel bulb, and parsnips

2 bulbs garlic, halved (you may also use the leftover skins from roasted garlic)

5 cups Muir Glen or San Marzano plum tomatoes, chopped (include tomato juice)

2 cups fresh parsley, stems and leaves, chopped

2 teaspoons whole black peppercorns

4 large bay leaves

several sprigs of fresh thyme

½ ounce dried mushrooms, such as porcini or shiitake,* optional

2 cups white wine, optional

6 quarts water

In a large stainless steel soup pot over medium-high heat, lightly brown the vegetables in the sesame oil. Add the remaining ingredients and cover with 3 inches of water. Bring to a boil, then reduce the heat and simmer the stock for 2 hours. Remove from heat and cool. Strain the stock through a large sieve into another pot. Using a measuring cup, portion the stock into Mason jars. Refrigerate and use within one week or freeze stock for up to three months.

---

*The dried mushrooms will add a nice earthy, meaty flavor to the stock.

Fish Stock

*Use white fish bones, such as halibut, for the stock. Bones from oily
fish, such as salmon or tuna, are too strong for a delicate stock.*

4 tablespoons cold-pressed sesame oil or coconut oil

4 cups yellow onions, chopped*

2 cups carrots, chopped

2 large garlic cloves, smashed

6 to 7 pounds fish bones, trimmings or heads (remove gills)

1 cup parsley, leaves and stems, chopped

1 to 2 large bay leaves

2 teaspoons organic lemon zest

2 cups dry white wine, optional

¼ cup white vinegar

6 quarts water

In a large stainless steel soup pot heat the sesame oil over medium-high heat. Add the vegetables and cook until soft. Add the fish bones, then add the rest of the ingredients and the water. Make sure the water covers the ingredients by 3 inches. Bring the stock to a boil and then reduce the heat. Simmer for 4 hours, skimming froth from the surface of the stock as needed. Remove from heat, cool, and then strain the stock through a large sieve into another pot. Using a measuring cup, portion the stock into Mason jars. Use within three days or freeze for up to two months.

---

*For an Asian version, omit the yellow onions and use scallions instead. Omit bay leaves and lemon zest and replace with 3 half-dollar-size slices of fresh ginger.

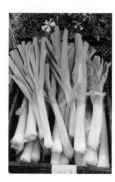

Oyster and Cauliflower Chowder
SERVES 8

This is a lighter but richly flavorful version of chowder. The homemade fish stock makes all the difference in this soup. Cauliflower adds a surprisingly delicious flavor, so you will not miss the potatoes.

4 ounces bacon,* finely diced

2 tablespoons ghee or cold-pressed sesame oil

3 cups sweet onions, chopped

2 cups thinly sliced leeks (white part only), rinsed of grit

2 teaspoons garlic, chopped

2 tablespoons coconut flour

6 cups fish stock (page 104)

2 sprigs fresh thyme

2 cups cauliflower, sliced ½-inch thick and cut into small cubes

2 cups organic pastured cream or coconut cream

⅓ cup dry sherry, optional

¼ teaspoon freshly ground black pepper

¼ teaspoon cayenne, optional

16 ounces fresh oysters or clam meat (add oysters to
    the soup just prior to serving)

salt and freshly ground pepper, to taste

Garnish: 4 teaspoons chopped Italian (flat leaf) parsley or chives

In a large sauté pan cook the bacon until crisp. Remove and set aside.

In a large stainless steel soup pot, heat the ghee or sesame oil. Then sauté the onions, leeks, and garlic until soft. Add the coconut flour and mix well, cooking for another 30 seconds. Add the fish stock and thyme and bring to a soft boil. Add the cauliflower, bring to a boil again, and reduce the heat to simmer. Continue cooking until the cauliflower is tender.

Just before serving, add the cream, sherry, salt, and pepper. Bring the soup to the boiling point again and drop in the oysters. As a variation, add 1 pound of baby spinach leaves to the soup just prior to serving. Cook the spinach until just wilted.

To serve, ladle the soup into large soup bowls and garnish with the chopped parsley or chives. Serve immediately.

---

*Try Beeler's or Llano Seco humanely raised bacon.

Summer Squash Soup with Mint Pesto

SERVES 8

Did you ever wonder what to do with all those summer squash in the garden? Well, this recipe with tasty mint pesto is the answer. When buying squash at the store make sure it is organic. By law organic also means not genetically modified.

The Soup

    4 tablespoons ghee or cold-pressed sesame oil

    1 medium sweet onion, thinly sliced

    ½ teaspoon sea salt

    2 pounds yellow or green summer squash, halved
      and thinly sliced

    2 carrots, thinly sliced

    4 cups chicken stock or vegetable stock (pages 102–3)

The Pesto

    1 cup fresh mint leaves

    ⅔ cup Italian (flat leaf parsley), leaves only

    2 scallions, chopped

    1 clove of garlic, chopped

    4 tablespoons pine nuts

    ¼ cup extra-virgin olive oil, more if needed

    1 teaspoon lemon juice

    pinch of sea salt and a twist of black pepper

For the soup: In a large, heavy-bottomed soup pot heat the ghee or sesame oil over medium heat. Add the onion to the pan with the salt and cook until soft. Add the squash, carrots, and stock, and bring the mixture to a simmer. Partially cover the pot and cook until the vegetables are tender, about 20 minutes. Remove the soup from the heat and cool about 15–20 minutes.

When the soup is cool enough, puree in small batches in a blender until very smooth. Return the soup to the same pot (after wiping it clean), and reheat.

For the pesto: Place all the pesto ingredients, except the olive oil, in the food processor and pulse several times until well incorporated. Then, with the motor running, slowly add the olive oil until the mixture forms a paste. Thin the mixture with a little water, if necessary, to achieve a smooth consistency. If you have leftover pesto, place it in a glass jar and cap with a little olive oil. Use the pesto within three days. If you put it on steamed veggies it won't last that long.

To serve: Ladle the soup into bowls and swirl a tablespoon of the pesto into the soup.

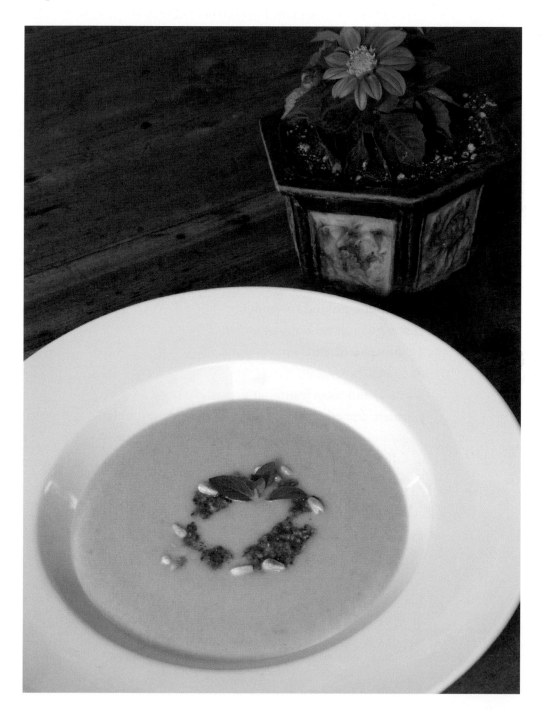

Santa Fe Chipotle Chili Soup with Lime Cream

SERVES 4 HEARTILY

When I lived in Santa Fe, I learned about the rich, smoky flavor of chipotle chilies. This easy-to-prepare soup is a hearty meal that will be at the top of the weekly request list.

The Soup

1 tablespoon canned chipotle chilies (use more at your own risk)

2 tablespoons water

2 yellow onions, finely diced

2 carrots, finely diced, optional*

2 stalks celery, finely diced

4 tablespoons cold-pressed sesame oil

4 cups chicken stock, divided (page 102)

1 teaspoon ground cumin

½ teaspoon ground coriander

½ teaspoon dried oregano

2 cups roasted chicken, chopped

juice of 2 limes

sea salt, and freshly ground pepper, to taste

Garnish: grated sheep's milk manchego or crumbled goat cheese, avocado slices, lime cream (recipe follows), lime slices, and sprigs of cilantro

The Lime Cream

1 cup Green Valley lactose-free sour cream, Capretta Rich and Creamy Goat Yogurt, or coconut cream

juice of 1 lime

---

*Some people cannot have root vegetables such as carrots because of the high sugar/starch content. I leave the decision as to its inclusion to you.

For the soup: In a blender puree the chipotle chilies and the water. Set aside.

In a large soup pot over medium heat sauté the onion, carrots, and celery in the sesame oil until soft. Add 1 cup of the stock. Cook, covered, until the liquid evaporates and the onions are soft and caramelized. Add the chili puree, remaining stock, cumin, coriander, and oregano. Simmer the soup for 5–10 minutes. Just before serving add the chicken, lime juice, salt, and pepper.

For the lime cream: Mix ingredients in a small bowl. Set aside until ready to use.

To serve: Ladle the soup into large soup bowls and garnish with the grated cheese, avocado slices, lime cream, and lime slices. Top with sprigs of cilantro.

Late-Summer Melon & Coconut Milk Soup

SERVES 4

This is a beautiful and wonderfully scented soup.

3 pounds very ripe and fragrant late-summer melon, divided

14 ounces coconut milk

1 to 2 jalapeños, seeded and finely diced

juice of 2 limes

zest of 1 lime

1 tablespoon garden basil leaves, chopped (Thai basil
    if you have it)

2 teaspoons microplaned ginger

1 tablespoon chopped mint

pinch of sea salt

Garnish: toasted unsweetened coconut (optional),
    sprigs of mint

Peel and seed the melon and cut the flesh into chunks, reserving ½ cup of finely diced melon.

In a food processor puree the melon. While the machine is running, pour in the coconut milk, jalapeño (add one and taste), ginger, mint, lime juice and zest, and salt. Chill the soup for several hours before serving.

To serve, pour the soup into small bowls and garnish with the toasted coconut and a sprig of mint.

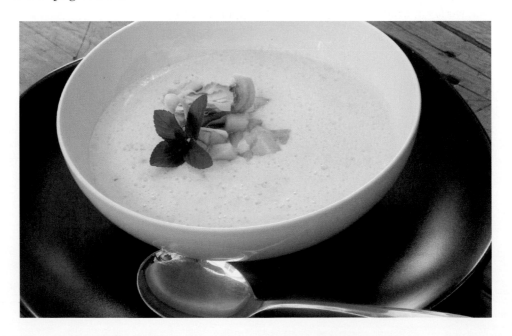

Curried Onion and Ginger Soup

SERVES 6

Caramelized onions, ginger, and curry mingle in this fragrantly rich soup.

2 tablespoons coconut oil

2 pounds Walla Walla, Vidalia, or another sweet
   onion

1½ teaspoons Madras curry powder

½ cup finely grated ginger, skin removed

1 small jalapeño, seeded and chopped

1 cup dry white wine

3½ cups coconut milk, divided into two portions

4 cups chicken or vegetable stock (pages 102–3)

2 tablespoons lime juice

½ teaspoon microplaned lime zest

sea salt and a twist of pepper to taste

Garnish: julienned basil leaves

In a large saucepan over medium heat, melt the coconut oil. Add the onions, curry powder, ginger, and jalapeño and cook until the onions are caramelized. Add the wine, stock, and half of the coconut milk. Simmer the mixture for 15 minutes. Remove from the heat and let cool about 10 minutes.

In a blender puree the soup in batches until very smooth. Return the soup to the saucepan and reheat, adding the other half of coconut milk, lime juice, and zest. Season the soup again with more salt and pepper to taste.

To serve, ladle the soup into bowls and garnish with the julienned basil leaves.

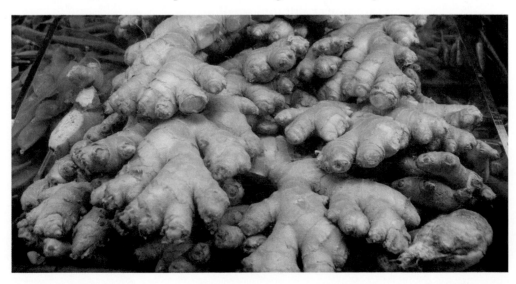

Thai Green Curry Chowder

SERVES 10

I think I like Thai green curry better than red curry. This soup is rich and complex and not too hot. You may substitute other vegetables in place of the bok choy if you prefer. If this recipe seems like too much, you can make the soup base and freeze some for a later use.

The Soup Base

4 tablespoons ghee, coconut oil, or cold-pressed
sesame oil

1 cup diced yellow onion

1 red or green Thai chili or jalapeño, seeded and
minced

¼ cup chopped garlic

2 cups dry white wine (optional) or add more water

2 cups coconut milk

4 tablespoons organic tomato paste

4 tablespoons Mae Ploy green curry paste, or to taste
(Mae Ploy contains shrimp paste)

4 cups homemade fish or vegetable stock (pages
103–4)

juice of 1 lime (more if desired)

The Soup Ingredients

¼ cup coconut oil

12 baby bok choy, trimmed of tough outer leaves

1 cup broccoli rabe, cut into very small pieces

1 cup cauliflower, cut into small pieces

8 ounces uncooked medium shrimp, peeled and
deveined, tails removed

8 ounces bay scallops

8 ounces enoki mushrooms, optional

3 tablespoons chopped mint

Garnish: cilantro sprigs, thin lime slices

For the base: In a large stainless steel soup pot over medium heat, melt the coconut oil. Add the onion, minced chili, and garlic and sauté until they are soft. Add the wine, coconut milk, tomato paste, curry paste, and stock; reduce the heat to low and simmer for 35–40 minutes. Add the lime juice. Adjust seasonings to taste.

For the soup ingredients: In a separate pot over medium heat, warm the coconut oil. Add the bok choy and sauté until it is still a bit crisp, not too soft (about 10 minutes). Add the broccoli rabe and cauliflower, shrimp, scallops, and enoki mushrooms and cook for 3–4 more minutes, stirring gently to mix well.

To finish the soup: Add the seafood/bok choy mixture to the soup base. Just before removing the soup from the heat, stir in the chopped mint.

To serve: Ladle into large soup bowls and garnish with the cilantro sprigs and lime slices. Serve immediately.

Hearty Vegetable Soup
with Basil Pesto

SERVES 10

*This soup is dinner in a bowl. Homemade pesto
is what makes this vegetable soup special.*

The Soup

2 tablespoons cold-pressed sesame oil

1 large yellow onion, diced

½ cup diced red bell pepper

2 large carrots, diced, optional

1 leek, white and light part only, washed and diced

3 tablespoons garlic, minced

½ small head green cabbage, thinly sliced

½ cup broccoli or cauliflower, cut into small pieces

1 bouquet garni (herb bundle) of 6 sprigs Italian (flat
  leaf) parsley, 6 sprigs thyme, and 2 bay leaves, tied
  with a string

6 to 8 cups chicken or vegetable stock (pages 102–3)

sea salt and freshly ground pepper, to taste

The Basil Pesto

3 to 4 garlic cloves, chopped

2 large bunches basil leaves (about 2 cups)

½ cup pine nuts or walnuts

a few drops of lemon juice

½ cup grated sheep's milk pecorino romano, or the
  Parmesan Cheese Substitute (page 152)

1 cup extra-virgin olive oil

For the soup: In a large stainless steel soup pot over medium heat, warm the sesame oil. Add the onion, bell pepper, carrots, leek, and garlic. Cook until the vegetables are tender. Add the cabbage and broccoli and the bouquet garni. Then, slowly add the stock while heating the soup, keeping it thick with the vegetables and not too thin. Season to taste with salt and pepper. When soup is hot remove from stove.

For the basil pesto: In the food processor, combine the garlic, basil, pine nuts, lemon juice, and the pecorino romano. Pulse several times to incorporate the ingredients. With the motor running, slowly add the 1 cup of olive oil, blending until the mixture is very smooth. Taste for seasonings.

If there is any leftover pesto, spoon it into a jar, cap with olive oil, and refrigerate for up to one week, or just freeze. Leftover pesto is great on cooked vegetables.

To serve: Ladle the soup into large soup bowls and top with a spoonful of the pesto. Pass some extra grated romano cheese.

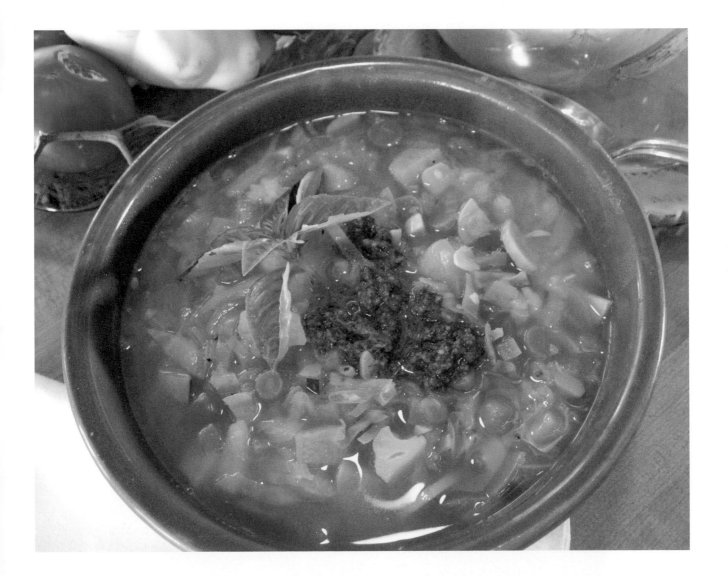

Spicy Heirloom Tomato Soup

SERVES 4

This soup makes a beautiful and zesty first course for a summer lunch or dinner. Heirloom tomatoes are fun to grow in your garden and are much less expensive than those purchased at the store.

1 pound ripe heirloom tomatoes or other organic tomatoes

2 tablespoons cold-pressed sesame oil

1 medium sweet onion, chopped

3 to 4 yellow or orange bell peppers, seeded and chopped, white pith removed

1 bay leaf

1 tablespoon fresh thyme leaves

1 teaspoon Chimayo chili powder or smoky Spanish paprika

2 cloves garlic, chopped

1 tablespoon organic tomato paste

1 teaspoon sea salt

1 teaspoon freshly ground pepper

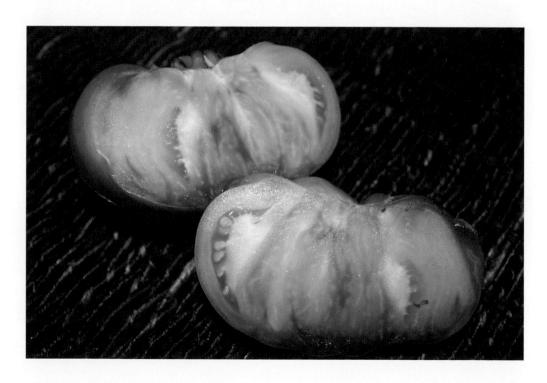

¼ cup water

4 cups chicken or vegetable stock (pages 102–3)

Garnish: slice of avocado, drizzle of extra-virgin olive
   oil, chopped basil leaves, chopped Italian parsley
   leaves

Cut an ✕ at the base of each tomato and drop it into a pot of boiling water for 2 minutes. Remove the tomatoes with tongs and set on a plate. When cool, cut in half and squeeze out the seeds, then remove the peel and dice the tomato.

In a large stainless steel soup pot heat the sesame oil over medium heat. Add the onions, peppers, bay leaf, thyme, and chili powder. Cook until the onion is soft, stirring a little, then add the garlic, tomato paste, salt, pepper, and the ¼ cup of water. Cook for 5 minutes and then add the tomatoes and the stock. Cover the soup and simmer for 25 minutes.

To serve, ladle the soup into bowls and garnish with the avocado slices, a drizzle of olive oil, and the chopped basil and parsley leaves.

Brazilian Shrimp Soup

SERVES 6 AS A MAIN COURSE

This soup is rich, complex, and very festive. If you cannot eat shellfish, substitute a white fish or diced, leftover roast chicken.* Serve the soup with a refreshing salad of mixed lettuces, orange or grapefruit sections, avocado, and a citrus-based dressing.

> 2 tablespoons coconut oil
> 1 large yellow or sweet onion, diced
> 5 cloves garlic, minced
> 2 small jalapeños, seeded and finely diced
> 2 tablespoons microplaned ginger
> 1 pound medium shrimp with shells[†] (reserve shells)
> 4 cups fish or vegetable stock (pages 103–4)
> 8 Muir Glen organic plum tomatoes, chopped
> 14 ounces coconut milk
> ⅔ cup almond butter
> ¼ cup fresh lime juice
> sea salt and a twist of black pepper, to taste
> ¼ cup chopped cilantro, leaves only
> Garnish: finely ground toasted almonds, cilantro
>   leaves, lime wedges

Remove the shells from the shrimp and set aside. In a large saucepan over medium heat, melt the coconut oil. Add the onion, garlic, chilies, ginger, and shrimp shells (shells only here, not the flesh). Cook the mixture over low heat until the onion is translucent. Add the stock and simmer for 15 minutes. Remove the stock from the heat, strain it, and return it to the saucepan. Then add the chopped plum tomatoes to the stock and simmer for another 10 minutes.

In the food processor, puree the coconut milk and almond butter until the mixture is smooth. Whisk this mixture into the stock. Then add the shrimp and the lime juice. Cook until the shrimp have just turned pink (about 3 minutes). Add salt and pepper to taste.

To serve, ladle the soup into bowls. Garnish with the finely ground almonds, cilantro leaves, and the lime wedges.

---

*If you are using chicken for the soup, use chicken stock.

[†]Check the Blue Ocean Institute website for safe shrimp: www.blueocean.org/programs, wseafood-search.

SALAD DAYS

All great salads have fresh, homemade salad dressings. I encourage you to use your favorite homemade dressings made with good oils, premium vinegars, freshly squeezed lemon juice, sea salt, and pepper. As a reminder, most commercially bottled dressings use genetically modified oils, artificial flavorings, preservatives, and hidden sources of gluten. If your kids are old enough they can learn to make their own favorite dressings. This way everyone has a chance to have the fun and responsibility of family food preparation.

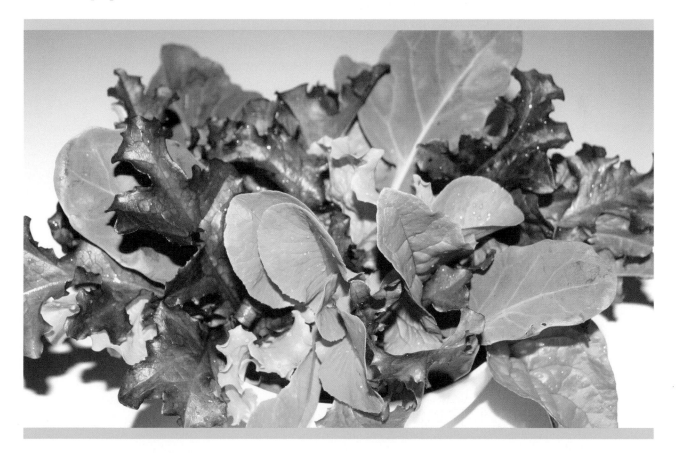

Family-Style Salad

If you don't want to think of a special salad to make for dinner, just put out your favorite organic lettuce mix and then prepare small bowls of diced celery, raw broccoli, cauliflower, sprouts, red bell pepper, and avocado and mushroom slices. Don't forget the jars of nuts and seeds. Let everyone concoct their own salad with their favorite dressing.

Blue Cheese Dressing

MAKES ABOUT 1 CUP

Spoon this dressing onto a wedge of chilled iceberg lettuce.

   2 tablespoons extra-virgin olive oil
   ¼ cup red onion, very thinly sliced
   1 tablespoon balsamic vinegar
   pinch of sea salt
   3 ounces Point Reyes Blue Cheese Crumbles (raw cow's milk)
      or raw sheep blue cheese or goat blue cheese*
   ¼ cup pastured cream or goat yogurt cream
   twist of pepper

In a bowl whisk together olive oil, onion, balsamic vinegar, and salt. In a food processor, blend the blue cheese and the cream or yogurt. Add the cheese mixture to the bowl of other ingredients and mix well. Refrigerate until ready to use.

---

*Some possibilities: Berger Basque raw sheep's milk cheese, Bleu du Bocage rare blue goat's milk cheese, and Roquefort Papillon, a raw sheep's milk blue cheese.

Citrus Vinaigrette

MAKES 3 OR MORE CUPS

Citrus vinaigrette is a refreshing choice to use when fruit is in the salad.
It's also great with a seafood salad.

¼ cup whole-grain mustard

1 cup freshly squeezed orange juice

¼ cup fresh lemon juice

¼ cup fresh lime juice

⅓ cup Champagne vinegar

2 tablespoons each chopped chervil and chives

1 teaspoon each organic lemon and lime zest

1 cup extra-virgin olive oil

sea salt and freshly ground pepper, to taste

In a bowl combine all ingredients, except olive oil, then slowly whisk in the oil. Season to taste with the salt and pepper.

Lemon Oregano Dressing

MAKES ABOUT 1½ CUPS

This dressing is excellent on a Mediterranean-style salad, grilled or
roasted vegetables, or on a seafood salad.

¼ cup fresh lemon juice

4 tablespoons balsamic vinegar

¼ cup fresh oregano leaves

2 cloves minced garlic

2 tablespoons capers, rinsed

¾ cup extra-virgin olive oil

sea salt and freshly ground pepper, to taste

Place ingredients in a blender and puree until well blended.

Poppyseed Dressing

MAKES 1½ CUPS

This dressing has a balance of sweet and tart and would complement a shrimp or crab salad with ripe summer fruit. Try the dressing as a party dip for fruit kebabs.

¾ cup Capretta Rich and Creamy Goat Yogurt, raw
  cream, or coconut cream
1 tablespoon poppy seeds
1 jalapeño, seeded and finely diced
½ cup fresh lime juice
¼ cup freshly squeezed orange juice
pinch of sea salt and a twist of pepper

Whisk together all the ingredients in a bowl. Season to taste.

Ranch Dressing

MAKES ABOUT 2 CUPS

Ranch dressing is an American classic, and this tasty recipe will take care of your hankering very nicely, but without all the additives in commercial ranch dressing. Use it as a vegetable dip for parties. You will never buy bottled ranch dressing again after you taste this one.

1 cup Homemade Mayonnaise (page 123)
1 cup pastured cream or coconut cream
1 teaspoon celery seed or 1 tablespoon celery leaves, minced
4 tablespoons chopped fresh parsley
4 tablespoons scallions, white and green parts, minced
1 teaspoon fresh oregano, minced, optional
2 teaspoons minced garlic
2 teaspoons onion powder
juice of ½ lemon
dash of cayenne
1 teaspoon sea salt and a twist of ground pepper

Place all the ingredients in a blender and puree until smooth. This dressing is best if used within a week.

Homemade Mayonnaise

MAKES 3 CUPS

*Because some of the dressing recipes call for mayonnaise,
it is essential that you make your own at home out of good oils.*

2 eggs, at room temperature
1 teaspoon Dijon mustard
3 tablespoons lemon juice or vinegar of your choice
pinch or two of sea salt
1 cup extra-virgin olive oil, avocado oil, or cold-pressed sesame
   oil (I like to use a blend of all three)

In a blender or food processor place the eggs, Dijon mustard, lemon juice or vinegar, and a pinch of sea salt. Turn on the blender and add the oil very slowly until the mixture emulsifies to the desired consistency. Check the seasoning for balance. You may want to add more sea salt, mustard, or lemon juice.

Homemade mayonnaise will keep for about one week in the refrigerator.

Variation: Caper Tarragon Mayonnaise

In addition to the recipe above, also add:

1 tablespoon drained capers
2 teaspoons chopped fresh tarragon

Variation: Red Pepper Mayonnaise

In addition to the recipe above, also add:

¼ to ⅓ cup roasted red bell peppers
½ teaspoon paprika or dash of Tabasco

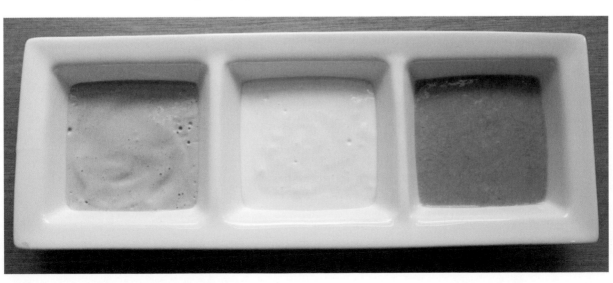

Roasted Garlic Vinaigrette

MAKES 1 OR MORE CUPS

The roasted garlic adds a mellowness to this yummy dressing.
It is a great accompaniment to almost any salad.

3 to 4 bulbs Roasted Garlic (page 85)
1½ tablespoons Dijon mustard
¼ cup rice wine vinegar
¾ cup extra-virgin olive oil
sea salt and a twist of pepper, to taste

Squeeze the roasted garlic into the blender, add the remaining ingredients, and puree until smooth.

Savory Green Salad

SERVES 4

This is a good everyday salad with big taste and lots of interest.

The Salad
4 cups savory greens, such as watercress, arugula,
   mizuna, or microgreens
4 Toasted Goat Cheese rounds (page 86)
Garnish: ½ cup chopped walnuts or pecans, 1 cup
   sunflower seed sprouts or another favorite sprout

The Dressing
1 tablespoon minced shallot
2 tablespoons Spanish sherry vinegar
1 tablespoon balsamic vinegar
¼ cup extra-virgin olive oil
1 tablespoon lemon juice
pinch of sea salt and a twist of pepper

In a small bowl whisk together the dressing ingredients.

In a large bowl toss the greens with the dressing. Arrange the greens on 4 salad plates. Place the toasted goat cheese on top of each salad and sprinkle with the pecans or walnuts. Garnish with the sprouts.

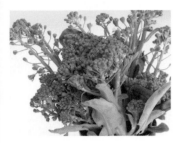

Broccoi Rabe and Feta Salad

SERVES 6

This salad makes a meal.

The Salad

2 pounds broccoli rabe, bottoms trimmed, cut into
  2-inch pieces

½ cup sliced red onion

¼ cup each fresh basil, cilantro and Italian (flat leaf)
  parsley, chopped

½ cup pine nuts, toasted

6 ounces Redwood Hill Farm Raw Goat Feta,
  crumbled

½ teaspoon sea salt and several twists of freshly
  ground pepper

Garnish: more feta if desired, organic cherry
  tomatoes, halved, Greek Kalamata Olives, drizzle
  of olive oil

The Dressing

2 tablespoons lemon juice

2 tablespoons Dijon or whole-grain mustard

1 tablespoon balsamic vinegar

4 tablespoons extra virgin olive oil

¼ teaspoon red pepper flakes

In a large pot of boiling water place the broccoli rabe and let it cook for 2–3 minutes, until softened and bright green. Drain the broccoli rabe and immediately plunge into ice water to stop the cooking. Remove the broccoli to a plate.

In a large bowl whisk together the lemon juice, mustard, balsamic vinegar, olive oil, red pepper flakes, and herbs. Add the cooked broccoli, red onion, feta, pine nuts, sea salt, and pepper. Keep folding all the ingredients together with a wooden spoon or rubber spatula until well combined.

To serve, portion the salad onto 6 salad plates. Garnish with more crumbled feta if desired, a drizzle of olive oil, and another twist of pepper. Surround the salads with the cherry tomatoes and olives.

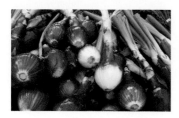

Salad of Grilled Vegetables with Feta Cheese

SERVES 6 TO 8

This salad would make a very hearty vegetarian entrée. You can also serve the salad with the Greek Lamb Kebabs (page 210).

The Vegetables

- 1 pound fresh asparagus, tough bottoms trimmed
- 4 zucchini, halved lengthwise
- 4 Japanese eggplants, halved lengthwise
- 4 vine ripened tomatoes, halved
- 2 red onions, sliced thick
- 8 large jalapeños, halved and seeded, optional
- 2 ripe avocados, cut in half, pit and skin removed
- ¼ cup cold-pressed sesame oil (for brushing on vegetables)
- 8 ounces Redwood Hill Farm Raw Milk Feta, crumbled, or another grated raw cheese
- ¼ cup fresh mint leaves chopped
- Garnish: additional crumbled feta, 1 cup Kalamata olives, your favorite greens (arugula is nice), toasted pine nuts, sprigs of mint

The Dressing

- 4 tablespoons extra-virgin olive oil
- 2 tablespoons aged balsamic vinegar
- 2 tablespoons fresh lemon juice
- 1 teaspoon red pepper flakes
- 1 teaspoon toasted ground cumin
- 1 teaspoon minced garlic
- pinch of sea salt and a twist of pepper

For the grilled vegetables: Heat the grill to medium hot. Place the vegetables on a sheet pan and brush liberally with four tablespoons of the sesame oil. Grill the asparagus, zucchini, onion slices, jalapeños, avocados, and tomatoes for about 5 minutes. Remove from grill and keep warm. Grill the eggplant for about 10 minutes or until fork tender. Remove all the vegetables to a cutting board and cut into attractive, bite-size pieces.

   For the dressing: Whisk together the balsamic vinegar, lemon juice, olive oil, red pepper flakes, cumin, salt, and pepper.

   To serve: Place a bed of greens on a large platter. Arrange the grilled vegetables on top. Spoon the dressing liberally over the top of the vegetables. Garnish the salad with more crumbled feta, the Kalamata olives, toasted pine nuts, and the mint. Give the salad a few twists of black pepper.

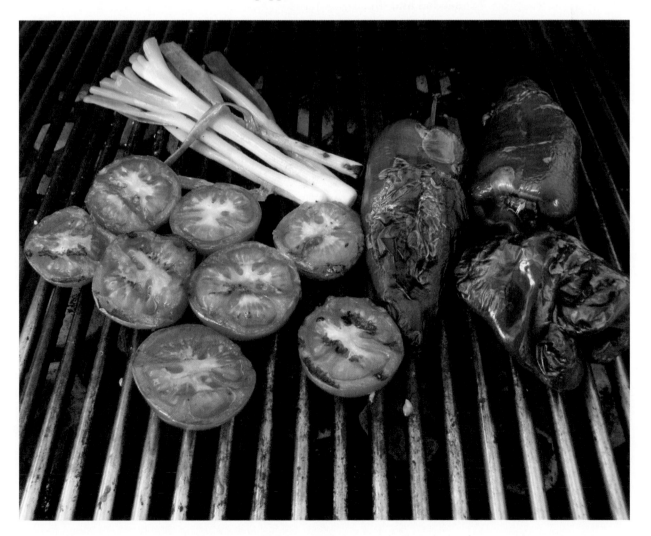

Barbecued Chicken Salad

SERVES 6

This salad is a simple, quick-to-make meal when you have leftover chicken. You can also use any combination of lettuces that you fancy. Leftover steak will also work in place of chicken. This is a family-friendly recipe.

The Salad

2 cups leftover roasted chicken, shredded

2 stalks celery, finely diced

1 red onion, finely diced

½ cup Mediterranean cucumber or English cucumber, seeded and diced

¼ cup toasted pecans, chopped

2 carrots, grated, optional

¾ cup grated cheese, such as Spanish manchego or raw cheddar

½ head Napa cabbage, thinly sliced

1 cup radicchio, thinly sliced

6 tablespoons Grilled Tomato Ketchup (page 153) or bottled organic chipotle sauce,* to taste

sea salt and freshly ground pepper, to taste

Garnish: ½ cup cilantro leaves, 12 to 16 organic cherry tomatoes, halved

The Dressing

1 clove of garlic, minced

1 teaspoon Dijon mustard

3 tablespoons red wine vinegar

1 teaspoon fresh thyme leaves

¾ cup extra-virgin olive oil

sea salt and freshly ground pepper, to taste

For the salad: In a large bowl place the shredded chicken. Add the diced celery, red onion, cucumber, toasted pecans, grated carrots, cheese, Napa cabbage, radicchio,

---

*Try Arizona Pepper's Organic Harvest Chipotle Habanero Pepper Sauce. Be careful!

and Grilled Tomato Ketchup. Sprinkle the ingredients with a pinch of salt and add a twist of pepper. Mix salad ingredients gently and thoroughly.

For the dressing: In a medium bowl whisk together all the dressing ingredients.

To serve: Arrange the salad ingredients on 6 plates. Whisk the dressing again and spoon it liberally over each salad. Garnish with the cilantro leaves and cherry tomato halves.

Pastured Egg Salad

SERVES 4

Egg salad is a childhood favorite. Serve on a bed of lightly dressed lettuce with some beautiful olives.

8 pastured or organic, free-range eggs

$^1/_3$ cup Homemade Mayonnaise (page 123)

3 scallions, white and light green parts, thinly sliced

1 tablespoon tarragon leaves, chopped

1 tablespoon flat-leaf parsley, chopped

1 tablespoon Dijon or whole-grain mustard

squeeze of lemon juice or to taste

pinch of sea salt and a twist of pepper

dash of cayenne

4 cups of your favorite lettuce

2 tablespoons extra-virgin olive oil

Garnish: 1 tablespoon chopped chives, ¼ cup thinly
    sliced radishes, your favorite olives

In a saucepan of cold water bring eggs to a boil. Boil for 2 minutes and then turn off the heat. Cover the pan and let the eggs sit for about 6 minutes. Place the eggs in cold water to cool, then peel.

In a bowl mash the eggs with a fork. Add the mayonnaise, scallions, tarragon, parsley, mustard, lemon juice, salt, pepper, and cayenne. Mix well and taste for seasoning balance. Add more mayonnaise if necessary.

In another bowl toss lettuce with the 2 tablespoons olive oil to coat.

To serve the salads, mound the lettuce onto 4 dinner plates. Spoon the egg salad onto the center of each mound. Garnish with the chopped chives, radishes, and olives.

Turkey Salad with Apple & Mint

SERVES 8

This easy salad is a great way to use leftover Thanksgiving turkey. It will feed the family the day after the holiday so you can relax. This is also a great buffet salad for a party. During the rest of the year, you can simply purchase and roast a turkey thigh.

The Salad

- 4 cups leftover turkey, shredded (leftover roast chicken or pork roast will also work)
- ½ cup toasted hazelnuts, walnuts, pecans, or pine nuts
- 1 cup organic apples (tart and crisp)
- ½ cup chopped celery
- ½ cup fresh mint, finely chopped
- 2 scallions, white and green part, thinly sliced on the diagonal
- 8 ounces organic lettuce mix or other favorite greens, such as baby arugula and watercress
- Garnish: Sprigs of mint

The Dressing

- ¾ cup extra-virgin olive oil
- ¾ cup freshly squeezed organic orange juice
- 2 tablespoons microplaned orange zest
- Stevita stevia, to taste
- 1 tablespoon Dijon mustard or whole-grain mustard
- ¼ teaspoon sea salt and a twist of fresh pepper

In a large bowl whisk together the olive oil, orange juice, orange zest, salt, and twist of pepper. Add the turkey, nuts, apples, celery, mint, and scallions. Toss well to mix dressing.

To serve, arrange 1 ounce (⅛ of the whole amount) of the lettuce on each plate. Top with the dressed salad mixture. Garnish with additional mint sprigs.

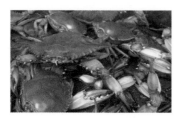

Crab and Grapefruit Salad with Microgreens & Herbs

SERVES 4

This easy-to-prepare salad is beautiful and wonderfully refreshing. Perfect for a luncheon!

1 large 1¾-pound red grapefruit

1 large 1¾-pound white grapefruit

6 tablespoons grapefruit juice

4 tablespoons extra-virgin olive oil

pinch of sea salt and a twist of pepper

½ cup fresh basil leaves, optional

½ cup fresh mint leaves, preferably from the garden

½ cup fresh tarragon leaves, removed from the stem

1 cup watercress or baby arugula

2 tablespoons minced chives or scallions, white part only

12 to 16 ounces cooked Dungeness crab meat (you can also use shrimp)

1 avocado, pit and skin removed, sliced

Garnish: ⅔ cup microgreens

Peel and segment the grapefruit by cutting between the sections with a sharp knife. Reserve 6 tablespoons of the juice.

In a small bowl whisk together the grapefruit juice, olive oil, salt, and pepper. Set the dressing aside.

Wash the herbs and greens gently and pat dry. Stack the basil leaves, roll into a cigar shape, and slice very thin. This is called a chiffonade. In a bowl combine all the herbs and greens (but not the microgreens for garnish) and the minced chives.

To serve, place the herbs-and-greens combination on 4 salad plates. Divide the grapefruit sections around the herbs. Place the crab on top of the greens. Spoon the grapefruit-juice dressing on top of each salad. Garnish the top of the salad with the microgreens and avocado.

Seafood Salad with Mangoes, Avocado & Meyer Lemon Vinaigrette

SERVES 4 AS AN ENTRÉE

Mangoes and avocados are gorgeous together. This fresh and lovely composed salad has two complementary dressings. You can also use slices of quickly seared tuna in the salad instead of crab or shrimp.

Meyer Lemon Vinaigrette

2 tablespoons Meyer lemon juice (or 1 tablespoon lemon juice and 1 tablespoon fresh orange juice)

zest of 1 Meyer lemon

¼ teaspoon sea salt and a twist of pepper

¼ cup extra virgin olive oil or cold-pressed sesame oil

The Salad

12 ounces (total weight) lightly cooked Dungeness crab and shrimp

8 ounces (total) baby arugula, watercress, or red oak leaf lettuce

1 ripe, firm mango, peeled, seeded, and diced

1 large, ripe avocado, peeled and diced

zest of 2 limes

Ginger Dressing

½ cup Homemade Mayonnaise (page 123; use sesame oil)

1 teaspoon microplaned ginger

1 teaspoon Coconut Secret Raw Coconut Aminos*

2 tablespoons Meyer lemon juice (or 1 tablespoon regular lemon juice and 1 tablespoon fresh orange juice)

For the Meyer Lemon Vinaigrette: In a small bowl whisk together the lemon juice, zest, salt and pepper.

   For the salad: In a medium bowl place the seafood and mix in 2 tablespoons of the vinaigrette. In another bowl gently toss the salad greens, the diced mangoes, avocado, and lime zest with the remaining vinaigrette.

---

*To replace tamari for those that cannot have gluten or soy foods.

For the ginger dressing: In a small bowl mix all the ingredients. Cover and chill until used.

To serve: To plate the salads divide the mango-lettuce mixture onto 4 plates, then top with the seafood mixture. Dot some of the ginger dressing on the salads or serve it on the side.

Sautéed Chicken Livers with Summer Greens

SERVES 4

Chicken livers are delicious and rich.
This salad could be lunch or dinner.

12 ounces organic chicken livers, preferably from
    pastured chickens
½ teaspoon sea salt and a twist of pepper
2 tablespoons ghee or cold-pressed sesame oil
3 tablespoons aged balsamic vinegar, divided
8 cups favorite summer greens (such as mesclun,
    baby arugula, and watercress)
4 tablespoons extra-virgin olive oil
1 tablespoon lemon juice

Place the chicken livers on a plate and sprinkle with the sea salt and pepper.

In a heavy-bottomed skillet heat the ghee or sesame oil to medium heat and cook the livers for 5–7 minutes or until brown on the outside but fairly pink inside. Take the pan off the heat and deglaze it with 2 tablespoons of balsamic vinegar. Stir the livers to coat with the vinegar.

In a large bowl toss the salad greens lightly with the extra-virgin olive oil, 1 tablespoon of balsamic vinegar, and lemon juice. Place the dressed greens on 4 salad plates.

Divide the livers onto the salads and spoon extra sauce from the pan over them. Pass the pepper grinder.

Caesar Salad
SERVES 8

Everyone loves Caesar salad, and this dressing is one of my standards from catering days. For a variation, if you don't like anchovies, you can use prepared horseradish. The dressing makes a fantastic dip for vegetables or party shrimp. It's also great on steamed or grilled vegetables. I love to have Caesar dressing in the refrigerator for a quick lunch. For an entrée salad, use about 3 ounces per person of cooked chicken, seafood, or steak. For nongluten croutons, use Lydia's Organics Sunflower Seed Bread or make your own croutons from the cookbook Everyday Raw *by Matthew Kenny or the cookbook* I Am Grateful: Recipes and Lifestyle of Café Gratitude *by Terces Engelhart.*

The Caesar Dressing
1¼ cups extra-virgin olive oil
1 tablespoon lemon juice
¼ cup red wine vinegar
3 egg yolks, preferably from pastured chickens
1 teaspoon minced garlic
1 tablespoon Dijon mustard
1 tablespoon aged balsamic vinegar,* optional
3 tablespoons chopped anchovies or anchovy paste
3 tablespoons sheep's milk pecorino romano, grated,
   or Parmesan Cheese Substitute (page 152)
pinch of sea salt and a twist of pepper
Garnish: grated romano, black pepper

The Salad
2 heads prewashed, organic romaine lettuce, chilled

For the dressing: In a large measuring cup whisk together the olive oil, lemon juice, and vinegar. In a blender combine the remaining dressing ingredients. While the blender is running, on medium speed, slowly add the oil, lemon juice, and vinegar mixture until the dressing is emulsified.

*Balsamic vinegar replaces Worcestershire sauce, which contains wheat, soy, and high fructose corn syrup.

For the salad: Chop the desired amount of the prewashed and chilled romaine lettuce leaves. The colder the better! Place the lettuce in a large bowl and add the dressing to liberally coat the leaves.

Serve the salad immediately. Garnish with more grated pecorino and black pepper.

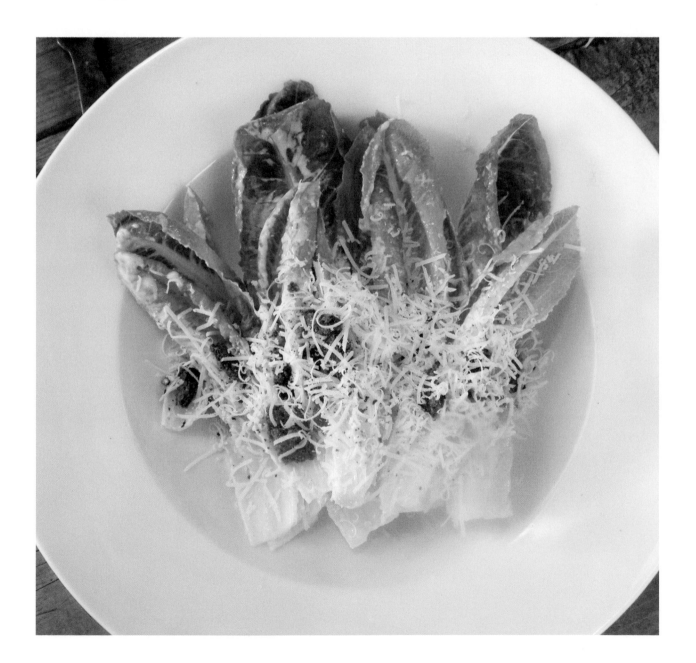

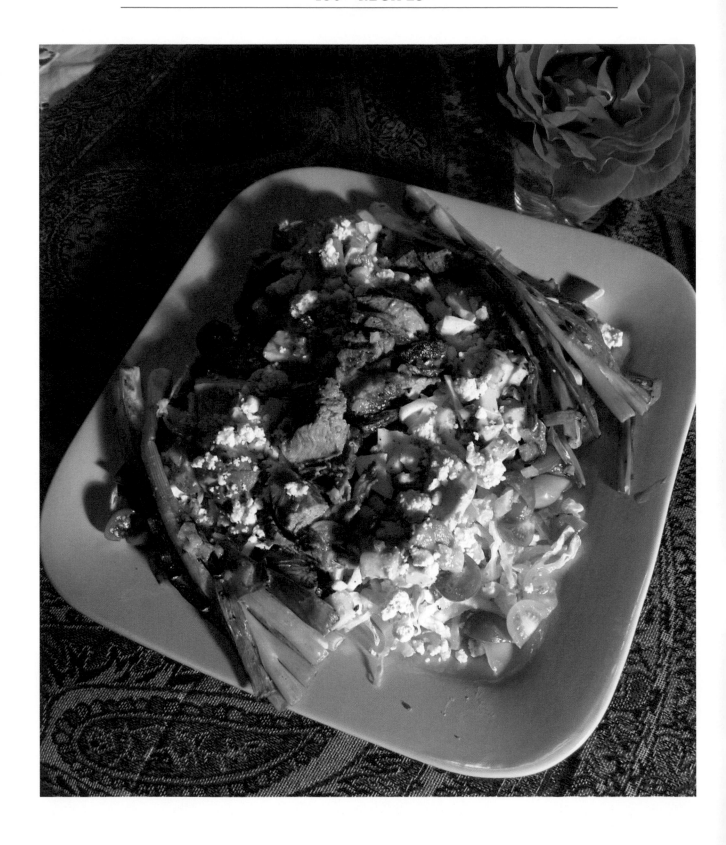

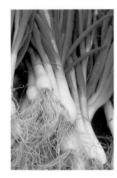

Colorful Cobb Salad

SERVES 4

Cobb salad makes a substantial meal, and you can use steak, chicken, or seafood to suit your preference. This salad will please your family or guests for a Sunday luncheon.

The Salad

8 ounces cooked steak, chicken, or seafood, cut into
   ½-inch cubes

4 hardboiled eggs, peeled and quartered

½ cup Pt. Reyes Blue Cheese Crumbles (raw cow's
   milk) or another raw blue cheese*

1½ cups diced ripe red or yellow tomatoes or organic
   cherry tomatoes, halved

8 cups mesclun mix or your favorite lettuce

1½ cups diced avocado

12 grilled or roasted scallions, room temperature and chopped

Garnish: 4 tablespoons chives cut into ½-inch pieces

The Cobb Dressing

1 minced shallot

⅓ cup lemon juice

1 cup extra-virgin olive oil

2 tablespoons minced chives

pinch of sea salt and a twist of pepper

First prep your ingredients and set them aside in separate bowls for ready assembly.

In a bowl whisk together the dressing ingredients, minced shallot, lemon juice, chives, and olive oil. Season with salt and pepper. Set aside.

In another bowl toss the diced tomatoes in 2 tablespoons of the dressing. In a large bowl toss the greens in half of the remaining dressing.

To serve, arrange the lettuce on 4 dinner plates. Place the salad ingredients in rows on top of the lettuce. Drizzle each salad with some of the remaining dressing. Garnish with the chives. Pass the pepper grinder.

---

*Other cheeses you might use: Berger Basque raw sheep's milk cheese, Bleu du Bocage goat's milk cheese, or Roquefort papillon raw sheep's milk blue cheese.

Beef Carpaccio Salad

SERVES 4

*This recipe works equally well with paper-thin slices of
roast turkey breast or smoked salmon.*

The Beef Carpaccio

12 ounces grassfed beef tenderloin

The Egg Cornichon

3 hard-boiled eggs, quartered

¾ cup radishes, minced

3 tablespoons capers, rinsed and chopped

3 tablespoons cornichons, minced

3 tablespoons fresh chives, chopped

The Vinaigrette

3 tablespoons fresh lemon juice

½ teaspoon sea salt and a twist of black pepper

7 tablespoons extra-virgin olive oil

6 ounces baby arugula

Garnish: 4 tablespoons microplaned sheep's milk
pecorino romano

For the beef carpaccio: Wrap the beef in plastic, and chill in freezer until firm, about 1 hour. Using a very sharp knife, cut the beef across the grain into ⅛-inch thick slices. Gently pound slices between pieces of waxed paper. Refrigerate the beef slices between the pieces of waxed paper for 1–2 hours.

For the egg-cornichon mixture: Force the hard-boiled eggs through a fine sieve into a small bowl. Add the radishes, capers, cornichons, and chives and mix the combination very gently.

For the vinaigrette: In a medium bowl whisk together the lemon juice, salt, and pepper. Slowly add the olive oil in a thin stream, whisking until the ingredients are emulsified.

To serve: First arrange the beef carpaccio (pounded beef slices) onto 4 large, chilled dinner plates. Drizzle all but 2 tablespoons of the vinaigrette over the meat, then sprinkle the egg-cornichon mixture on top.

Add the arugula to the bowl with the remaining 2 tablespoons of the vinaigrette.

Toss the greens with the 4 tablespoons of the grated pecorino romano. Mound the salad in the center of each plate on top of the carpaccio. Garnish with the chopped chives. Pass the pepper grinder if desired.

Japanese Salad

SERVES 6

This is a very nourishing entrée salad.

The Japanese Vinaigrette

  3 tablespoons Coconut Secret Raw Coconut
      Aminos,* or to taste
  3 tablespoons sesame oil (you can use toasted
      sesame oil)
  2 to 3 tablespoons seasoned rice wine vinegar
  3 tablespoons warm water

The Salad

  3 ounces per person leftover cooked chicken,
      seafood, or rare steak, chopped
  1 tablespoon pickled ginger
  2 carrots, peeled and cut into matchsticks
  1 small head radicchio, thinly sliced
  2 to 3 scallions, white and green part, sliced on the diagonal
  2 sheets nori, cut into thin strips, optional
  Garnish: 2 to 3 tablespoons toasted sesame seeds

For the Japanese vinaigrette: In a bowl large enough to hold the following salad ingredients, whisk together the coconut aminos, sesame oil, rice wine vinegar, and warm water.

  For the salad: Add the cooked meat or seafood, carrots, scallions, pickled ginger, and nori strips to the Japanese Vinaigrette. Toss well.

  To serve: Place the thinly sliced radicchio on the plates. Divide the dressed salad mixture onto each plate. Garnish the salads with the toasted sesame seeds.

---

*The aminos replace white miso for those who cannot consume foods containing soy.

Green Goddess Salad

SERVES 8

Green Goddess Dressing is as delicious as it is beautiful.
Use on cold, cooked vegetables as well as salad. This salad makes a meal.

The Salad

8 ounces favorite salad greens, such as romaine,
frisee, arugula, mesclun, or oak leaf

3 ounces per person, cooked chicken, steak or
seafood, finely chopped

2 to 3 Persian cucumbers or 1 English cucumber,
sliced lengthwise and then cut on the diagonal

1 small basket organic cherry tomatoes, halved

½ cup radishes, thinly sliced

Garnish: 3 tablespoons chopped chives

The Green Goddess Dressing

Makes about 2 cups

½ ripe avocado

1 large clove garlic, minced

2 tablespoons anchovy paste

1 large scallion, white and green parts, chopped

3 tablespoons tarragon leaves, chopped

2 tablespoons cilantro leaves, chopped

1 tablespoon basil leaves, chopped

¼ cup Italian (flat leaf) parsley, chopped

3 tablespoons lemon juice

3 tablespoons white wine vinegar

¾ cup extra-virgin olive oil

¼ cup Capretta Rich and Creamy Goat Yogurt, raw
cream, or coconut cream

sea salt and freshly ground pepper, to taste

For the Green Goddess Dressing: In a food processor, puree all the ingredients except the salt and pepper, olive oil, and yogurt. With the motor running, slowly add the olive oil until mixture is well incorporated. Remove the ingredients to a bowl and whisk in the yogurt. Season with salt and pepper, to taste.

To serve the salad: Arrange the greens, vegetables, and your selection of chicken, steak, or seafood attractively on large plates. Spoon the Green Goddess Dressing over the salads. Garnish with the chives.

Heirloom Tomato Caprese Salad

SERVES 6

For this classic Italian salad use fresh mozzarella di bufala, *which has a very creamy texture. Heirloom tomatoes make a beautiful presentation on the plate. For authentic flavor, the tomatoes you use should be just picked from the garden or purchased from the farmers' market. The better tasting the tomato, the better the salad!*

> **18 to 24 slices heirloom tomatoes (3 to 4 slices per salad)**
> **12 ounces (2 ounces per salad) mozzarella di bufala cheese (mozzarella made with buffalo milk)***
> **½ cup extra-virgin olive oil**
> **18 fresh basil leaves (tender leaves are best)**
> **Garnish: aged balsamic vinegar, Celtic Flower of the Ocean sea salt or Maldon sea salt (very light flakes), freshly ground pepper**

Arrange the tomatoes on 6 salad plates. Cut the mozzarella into attractive slices and overlap with the tomato slices. Arrange the basil leaves between the slices of tomatoes and mozzarella.

Drizzle the olive oil evenly over each salad and sprinkle with balsamic vinegar. Celtic Flower of the Ocean or Maldon sea salts are for finishing, so sprinkle on the salads for sparkle. Add a grind of pepper.

---

*Buffalo milk is A2 casein, but don't make this recipe if you are casein intolerant.

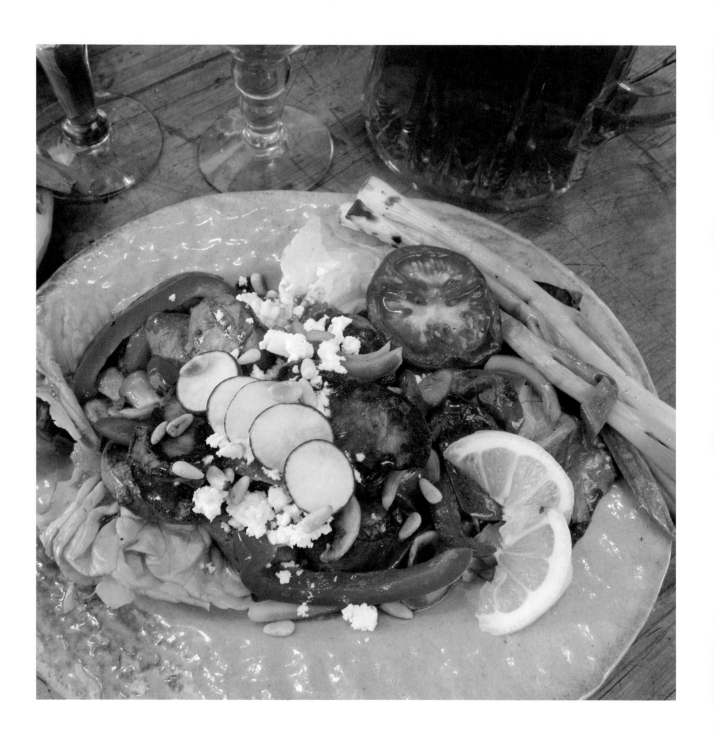

Chicken Sausage Salad

SERVES 2

I made this quick salad one day when I was visiting my daughter
Shannon and her husband, Anthony, in the Bay Area.

2 organic chicken sausages, chopped (Bruce Aidells
   or AmyLu)

2 tablespoons cold-pressed sesame oil

2 large handfuls organic spinach leaves

1 tablespoon balsamic vinegar

1 tablespoon lemon juice

2 large handfuls of your favorite lettuces

2 ounces Redwood Hill Raw Goat Feta or another
   grated raw cheese

Garnish: drizzle of extra-virgin olive oil, ½ cup
   organic cherry tomatoes, halved, sliced Persian
   cucumber, some favorite olives, toasted pine nuts,
   fresh pepper

In a large skillet, heat the sesame oil to medium-hot. Place the chopped sausage in the pan and begin to brown. Add the handfuls of spinach and begin to wilt, adding the balsamic vinegar and lemon juice. Toss ingredients well. Remove skillet from heat.

Place the salad greens in a large bowl. Toss with a drizzle of olive oil and a few drops of balsamic vinegar, to taste. Remove the greens to 2 large plates.

Divide the warm sausage/spinach salad mixture on top of the lettuce and top with the crumbled feta. Garnish the salads with another drizzle of olive oil, the cherry tomatoes, cucumber, olives, and pine nuts. A couple grinds of fresh pepper will finish the salads nicely.

Grilled Mexican Steak Salad
with Chipotle Chili Dressing

SERVES 4

Chipotle chilies are hot and smoky and make a spicy, flavorful dressing for this salad. You will find find chipotle chilies in small cans in the Mexican section at the grocery store. You may add more to this recipe if you like the heat turned up.

The Chipotle Chile Dressing

1 cup Homemade Mayonnaise (page 123) or Capretta
   Rich and Creamy Goat Yogurt
2 tablespoons extra-virgin olive oil
juice of 1 lime
1 teaspoon minced garlic
1 teaspoon canned chipotle chilies, pureed (taste for
   heat)
pinch of sea salt and a twist of pepper

The Salad

12 to 16 ounces grilled grassfed flank steak or sirloin
   (grilled chicken will also work)
1 large red onion, skin removed and sliced into thick
   rings
sea salt and freshly ground pepper
sesame oil for grilling
4 large garden tomatoes, cut in half and brushed with
   sesame oil
1 large head organic romaine lettuce, chopped
Garnish: avocado slices (½ avocado per person),
   ½ cup chopped cilantro leaves, ½ cup toasted
   pumpkin seeds or pine nuts

For the chipotle dressing: Blend the dressing ingredients together in the food processor or blender. Check for balance of flavors. Set aside.

For the salad: Place the chopped romaine in a large bowl. Refrigerate until ready to assemble the salad.

In a bowl mix the onion slices with some sesame oil to coat, season with a little salt and pepper. Brush the oil on the tomatoes and again season with salt and pepper. Brush the sesame oil on the flank steak and season both sides with salt and pepper.

With the grill turned to high, grill the steak to rare or medium rare. At the same time place the tomatoes, cut side down, on the grill and cook until well seared but not mushy. Also grill the onion slices on both sides.

When the steak, tomatoes and onions are done, remove from the grill to a platter and let cool for 5 minutes. On a cutting board, slice the steak very thin.

To serve the salad: Divide the chilled romaine onto 4 large plates. Arrange the grilled onions and tomatoes around the romaine and then top the salad with the thin slices of steak. Garnish the salads with the avocado slices, chopped cilantro, and toasted pumpkin seeds. Drizzle the salads with some of the chipotle dressing and pass the rest.

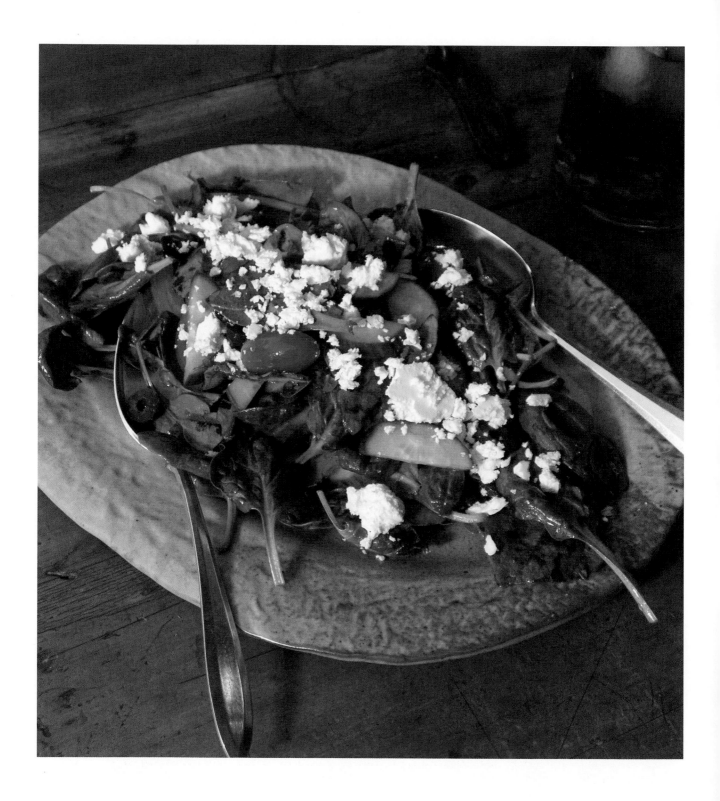

Mediterranean Spinach & Feta Salad with Lemon Dressing

SERVES 6

This classic salad is very fast to make. What makes it even more special is the Coriander Marinated Olives. The traditional Kalamata olives also work very well with this salad.

The Salad

12 ounces baby spinach leaves

6 ounces Redwood Hill Farm Raw Milk Feta, crumbled

2 to 3 ripe organic tomatoes cut into wedges or 1 cup organic cherry tomatoes, halved

2 to 3 small Persian or Mediterranean cucumbers,* sliced on the diagonal

1 red onion, skin removed and sliced into very thin rings

Garnish: The Coriander Marinated Olives (page 88) and lemon wedges

The Mediterranean Lemon Dressing

juice of 1 lemon

6 tablespoons extra-virgin olive oil

pinch of sea salt and a freshly ground pepper

In a small bowl whisk together the lemon juice and olive oil. Season with salt and pepper. Feta cheese is salty so you won't need much salt.

In a large bowl place the spinach and the feta cheese. Pour the lemon dressing over the spinach/feta mixture and gently toss until spinach is well coated.

To serve, place the spinach salad mixture on large plates with the tomatoes, red onion rings, and cucumbers. Garnish the salad with the coriander olives. Drizzle more olive oil if desired. Pass the pepper grinder.

---

*Persian or Mediterranean cucumbers are available at Trader Joe's, Whole Foods Market, and other markets.

Thai Salad with Spicy Ginger Dressing

SERVES 6

This salad is a whole meal. The dressing is exceptional and can also be used as a marinade for flank steak, chicken, or fish. You can prepare the salad as described here, or you can offer all the ingredients in separate bowls, buffet style, and let your guests have the fun of creating their own salads.

The Spicy Ginger Dressing (makes 2 cups or more)

¾ cup seasoned rice wine vinegar

1 cup cold-pressed sesame oil

¼ cup Coconut Secret Raw Coconut Aminos,* or to taste

juice of 1 lime (more if you like)

2 tablespoons minced garlic

4 tablespoons microplaned ginger

1 teaspoon red pepper flakes

1 jalapeño, seeded and finely diced

The Salad

½ head Napa cabbage, thinly sliced

2 cups cooked chicken, steak, or seafood, sliced thin or chopped

2 bell peppers (variety of colors), seeded and cut into matchsticks

2 carrots, peeled and cut into matchsticks, optional

1 bunch green onion, white and green parts, sliced on the diagonal

1 cup organic cherry tomatoes, halved

1 cup mung bean or sunflower seed sprouts

enoki or other fresh mushrooms, sliced

1 cup cilantro leaves, chopped

Garnish: 1 cup roasted macadamia nuts, finely chopped, 1 cup cilantro leaves

---

*Coconut aminos replace tamari for those who cannot consume soy or gluten foods.

For the dressing: In a bowl whisk together all the dressing ingredients. This dressing keeps well in the refrigerator.

For the salad: In a large bowl toss the thinly sliced Napa cabbage in "some" of the dressing, to just coat.

To serve the salad: Arrange the cabbage on a large platter. Scatter the cooked chicken, steak, or seafood on top of the cabbage. Artistically arrange the bell pepper, carrots, scallions, tomatoes, and mushrooms around the perimeter of the salad, then scatter the sprouts on top. Spoon some of the remaining dressing on top of the salad. Garnish with the macadamia nuts and the cilantro leaves. Pass more dressing if desired.

Mexican Cole Slaw
with Chipotle-Lime Dressing

SERVES 4

This is a unique version of a favorite. Make sure to dress the cold salad ingredients just before serving so that everything stays crunchy. The toasted almonds make this cole slaw unusual. Serve with fish tacos or grilled steak.

The Cole Slaw

- ⅓ cup almonds, chopped
- 1 teaspoon ghee
- 5 cups white cabbage, very thinly sliced (you may use white and red cabbage)
- 1 red bell pepper, seeded and very thinly sliced
- 1 organic apple, cored, quartered, and very thinly sliced
- 2 scallions, white and green parts, very thinly sliced on the diagonal
- Garnish: cilantro leaves, optional

The Chipotle-Lime Dressing

- ½ cup Homemade Mayonnaise (page 123)
- ¼ cup Capretta Rich and Creamy Goat Yogurt, raw cream, or coconut cream
- juice of ½ lime
- 1 teaspoon canned chipotle chili, pureed, or bottled chipotle sauce*
- Stevita stevia, to taste, if a little sweetness in the dressing is desired

For the salad: Heat the ghee on medium high in a small skillet. Add the almonds and sauté until light brown and fragrant. Immediately remove them from the pan.

Place all the salad ingredients in a large bowl and refrigerate until ready to dress.

For the chipotle dressing: whisk the ingredients together in a small bowl. Refrigerate until ready to dress the salad.

To serve: Just before serving toss the dressing into the salad ingredients and toss well. Garnish with the cilantro leaves.

---

*Try the Arizona Peppers Organic Chipotle-Habanero Pepper Sauce. But be careful!

CONDIMENTS AND SAUCES

Homemade sauces and condiments are not only healthier, they are also much tastier than store-bought versions. Everyone in your family will have a favorite condiment to make mealtime more interesting. Commercial condiments and sauces usually contain ingredients that should be avoided, such as soy, corn, and canola oils that are mostly genetically modified. These products also contain high fructose corn syrup, hidden gluten ingredients, toxic preservatives, and artificial flavors. Many reasons to make your own!

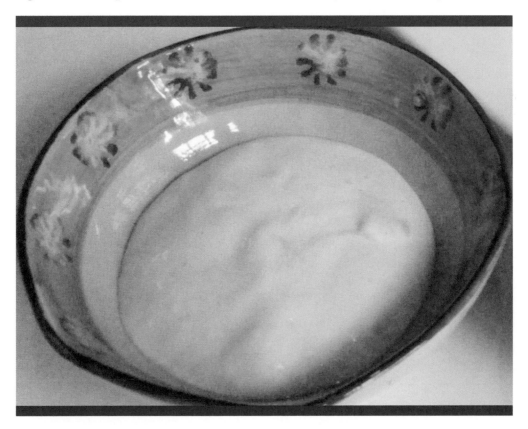

Parmesan Cheese Substitute

*Nora Gedgaudas gave me this suggestion for a parmesan cheese substitute,
and I think it works very well. Make a batch and keep it in the fridge
for a topping on salads and veggies. You can even use it in place of cheese
when making Caesar salad dressing or a pesto.*

1 tablespoon ghee
1 cup pine nuts or chopped walnuts
½ cup nutritional yeast
1 tablespoon Maldon sea salt*

In a small sauté pan, heat the ghee. Add the nuts and fry them until golden brown.
Be careful not to burn! Place the nuts in a food processor and pulse them until they're
finely chopped. Remove them to a bowl and add the nutritional yeast and Maldon salt.

Garlic Aioli

*Aioli is a luxurious, very garlicky sauce for steamed vegetables or grilled vegetables.
You can use aioli instead of mayonnaise. For a variation use Roasted Garlic
(page 85) to make the aioli. It will add a mellower flavor.*

6 cloves garlic, chopped
2 tablespoons sherry vinegar
2 eggs
1 tablespoon Dijon mustard
1 teaspoon sea salt and a twist of black pepper
½ cup extra-virgin olive oil
½ cup cold-pressed sesame oil

In a blender combine all the ingredients except the oils. Turn the blender on low to
start, then turn it up to high and slowly add the oils until they emulsify. Taste the
aioli and adjust the seasonings as necessary. For a variation, substitute lemon juice
for sherry vinegar. You can also add herbs, such as tarragon, or, seeded and minced
jalapeños if you want a spicy aioli.

---

*Maldon salt is a light, flaky salt from England. It has an especially clean taste. If you use another sea
salt, then use less, perhaps 1 teaspoon.

Grilled Tomato Ketchup

MAKES ABOUT 1 CUP

Making your own ketchup is fun. Most bottled ketchups, barbecue sauces,
and condiments have a high fructose corn syrup, MSG, and gluten.
Read labels and steer clear of these products.

small amount of cold-pressed sesame oil for brushing
   on the veggies
4 ripe, organic whole Roma tomatoes
1 small red onion, peeled and quartered
1 large jalapeño
2 tablespoons organic, unfiltered, apple cider vinegar
Stevita stevia, to taste, if you like a little sweeter flavor
1 tablespoon Dijon or whole-grain mustard or
   creamed horseradish
1 tablespoon fresh lime or lemon juice
¼ cup cilantro leaves, optional

Turn the grill up to high. Brush the tomatoes, onion, and jalapeño with the sesame oil, then grill or broil until lightly charred.

   In a food processor combine the cider vinegar, stevia, mustard or horseradish, and lemon juice. Pulse until the sauce is chopped and looks chunky. At this point, you can add the optional cilantro.

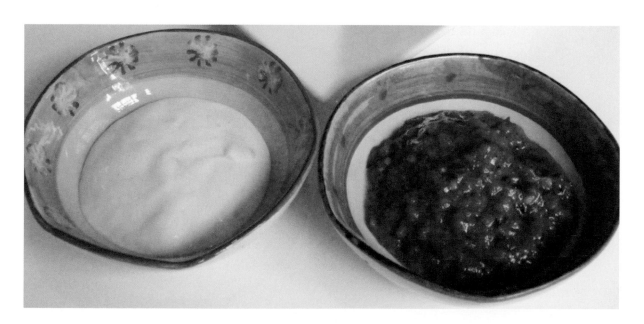

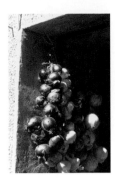

Rich and Spicy Italian Tomato Sauce

MAKES ABOUT 3 QUARTS

This rich tomato sauce is my version of the tomato sauce that one of my catering clients from Florence, Italy, used to make. She prepared huge batches of the sauce every summer with tomatoes from her garden. You can use this sauce when you make meatballs, or use it as a sauce for grilled chicken or fish. It's also great as a sauce for Roasted Vegetable Napoleons (page 158). This is my favorite tomato sauce.

3 pounds ripe organic tomatoes, peeled, seeded, and chopped

¼ cup cold-pressed sesame oil

1 large onion, minced

1 leek, rinsed of any grit, trimmed, and minced

1 whole bulb garlic, peeled and minced

2 jalapeños, seeded and minced

1 teaspoon red pepper flakes

3 celery ribs, trimmed and minced

½ cup fresh basil leaves, chopped

2 tablespoons fresh oregano leaves, chopped

½ cup dry red wine, optional

4 ounces pastured butter or Meyenberg Goat Milk Butter

sea salt and freshly ground pepper, to taste

To peel the tomatoes bring a large pot of water to a boil. Plunge the tomatoes in the boiling water until the skin just splits. Remove immediately to a platter and cool. When cool enough slice the tomatoes in half and squeeze the seeds out. Remove the skin with a paring knife and then chop the tomatoes.

In a heavy-bottomed pot heat the oil to medium high. Add the onion, leek, celery, and garlic and sauté until very caramelized. Add the jalapeños and red pepper flakes and cook for 1 minute longer.

Add the tomatoes, herbs, and red wine. Reduce heat to a simmer. Cook very slowly for about 1–1½ hours, stirring as needed. Toward the end of the cooking time, whisk in the butter, salt, and pepper. Cook for another 30 minutes to meld the flavors. Remove the sauce from the heat and let cool.

When the sauce is cool enough puree it in the food processor. If you want a very smooth textured sauce press the solids through a sieve. I think it's fine just the way it is.

Tapenade

MAKES APPROXIMATELY 3 CUPS

This traditional French condiment is great on grilled fish or with roast leg of lamb or grilled chops. Normally tapenade is served with buttered croutons; however, you may use the Lydia's Seed Bread or make your own crackers for a party. A dab of tapenade would dress up deviled eggs.

3 cups pitted Kalamata or Niçoise olives
2 tablespoons capers, rinsed
1 tablespoon anchovy paste or 2 salt-packed anchovies
½ cup toasted pine nuts or walnuts, finely chopped
1 garlic clove, minced
1 tablespoon fresh basil, chopped
1 tablespoon Italian (flat leaf) parsley, chopped
extra-virgin olive oil, as needed
pinch of cayenne or a twist of black pepper

Place all the ingredients—except the olive oil—in the bowl of a food processor. While pulsing the processor, drizzle the olive oil into the mixture and continue to pulse until the ingredients are very finely chopped. Add a pinch of salt if necessary, but taste the mixture as olives tend to be salty. The tapenade is now ready to serve.

Store the tapenade in jars in the refrigerator capped with a little olive oil. It should keep this way for several weeks.

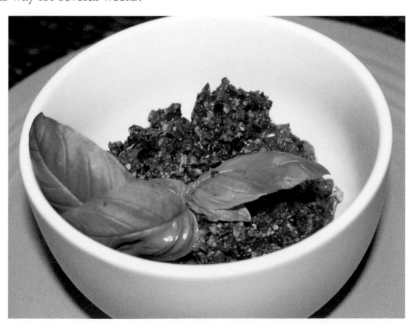

Very Green Herb Sauce

MAKES ABOUT 3 CUPS

This is a vibrant sauce for grilled chicken or fish. It's also a very pretty party dip for raw vegetables.

2 tablespoons organic apricot fruit puree (no added sugar)

4 cloves garlic, chopped

2 scallions, white and green part, finely chopped

1½ cups cilantro leaves, no stems

½ cup basil leaves

½ cup parsley leaves

½ cup tarragon, optional

½ cup pine nuts

¼ cup lemon juice

pinch of cayenne

sea salt and a twist of pepper

1 cup cold-pressed sesame oil

Place all ingredients—except sesame oil—in a food processor. With the motor running, gradually add the oil until the mixture is thick and creamy. Use immediately or store in a jar in the fridge. The sauce will keep for about three days.

EAT YOUR
VEGETABLES!

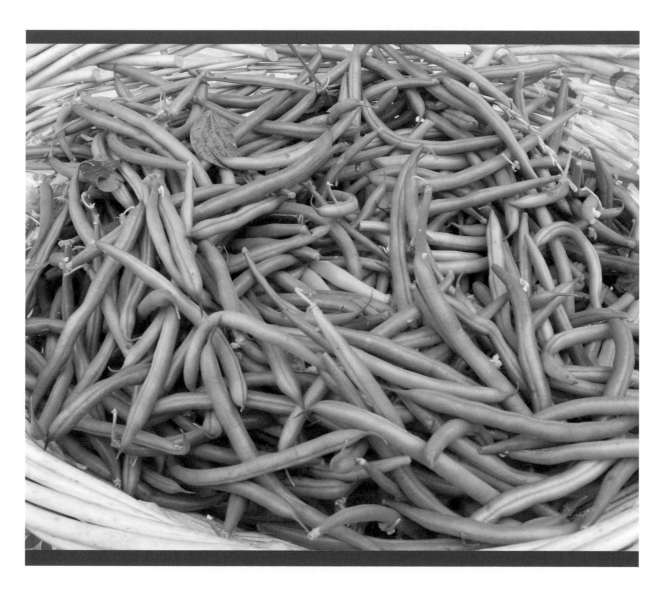

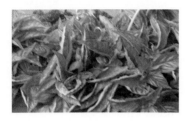

Roasted Vegetable Napoleons with Basil Pesto

SERVES 4

My Napa Valley catering company, The Best of Everything, served these gorgeous vegetable napoleons. They are great for lunch or as a first course. For lasagna without the pasta, you can drape them with the Rich and Spicy Italian Tomato Sauce (page 154).

The Pesto

3 to 4 garlic cloves, chopped

1 to 2 bunches basil leaves (about 2 cups)

½ cup pine nuts or walnuts

a few drops of lemon juice

½ cup grated sheep's milk pecorino romano or
    Parmesan Cheese Substitute (page 152)

1 cup extra-virgin olive oil

The Marinade

⅔ cup extra-virgin olive oil

⅓ cup balsamic vinegar

2 cloves garlic, minced

The Vegetables

4 3-inch-diameter portobello mushrooms

2 small eggplants, sliced about 1½ inches thick (8
    slices total)

4 ripe tomato slices, ½ inch thick

4 red onion slices, ½ inch thick

1 zucchini, trimmed and cut lengthwise into 4-inch-
    long slices

1 large red bell pepper, trimmed, seeded, and cut
    into 4 equal pieces

your favorite cheese, such as manchego, goat cheese,
    or raw jack, one slice for each napoleon, optional

1 to 2 bunches fresh garden basil, for placing in
    between the layers of vegetables

sea salt and a twist of pepper

Garnish: additional leaves of basil, olive oil for
drizzling

Preheat the oven to 400 degrees.

For the pesto: In a food processor, combine the garlic, basil, pine nuts, lemon juice, and pecorino romano. Turn on the processor and slowly pour in the olive oil adding more oil if necessary until the mixture is smooth. Taste the pesto and add a little salt, if necessary. Remove the pesto to a bowl, cap with a little olive oil, cover, and set aside.

For the marinade and vegetables: First mix the marinade in a small bowl. Brush the vegetables liberally with the marinade on both sides. Place the vegetables on a stainless steel sheet pan and lightly sprinkle with salt and pepper. Roast the vegetables in the oven until soft, turning once with a wide spatula.

To assemble: Set out 4 dinner plates. Beginning with the portobello mushroom, stack the vegetables, placing the basil leaves in between the layers. If you are using the cheese, place it in the middle of the napoleon. Drizzle the pesto around the perimeter of the napoleon and add a few drops of olive oil to make it glisten. Garnish with additional basil leaves.

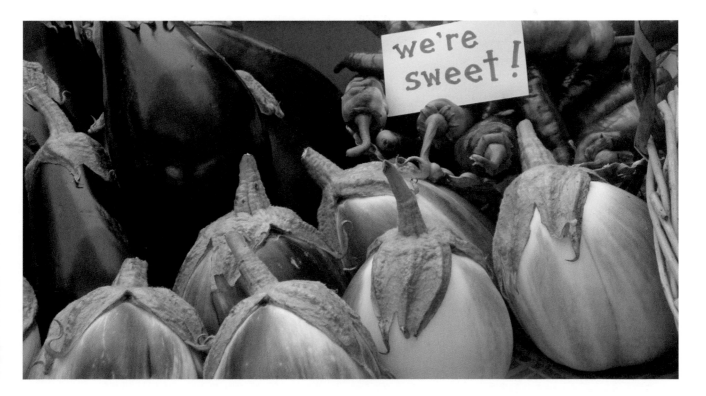

Cauliflower Rice

SERVES 4

*Easy, easy, easy! You can use Cauliflower Rice with any entrée that
you would normally serve with rice. I actually like it better than rice,
and I think your kids will too.*

1 large head cauliflower
2 to 3 tablespoons pastured butter, ghee, or cold-
    pressed sesame oil
1 small yellow onion, finely pulsed in a food
    processor
sea salt and freshly ground pepper, to taste

In a food processor, pulse the raw cauliflower until it resembles grains of rice.

In a large sauté pan, heat the butter, ghee, or sesame oil. Add the onion and sauté it
until translucent. Add the processed cauliflower, salt, and pepper and mix thoroughly
with the onion. Cover the pan, add a few tablespoons of water, and continue to cook
the mixture 5–10 minutes or until the cauliflower is softened. It is now ready to serve.

For variations, add some of your favorite fresh herbs or spices.

Sautéed Broccoli Rabe with
Pecorino Romano

SERVES 6

*Broccoli rabe is more expensive than regular broccoli, but it's very tender
and delicious, so for this dish, it's well worth the price. This is a good way
to get kids of all ages to like vegetables.*

4 tablespoons cold-pressed sesame oil, divided
½ small onion, cut in half and thinly sliced
4 cloves garlic, minced
½ teaspoon red chili flakes
2 bunches broccoli rabe, ends trimmed about 1 inch
2 tablespoons water
1 pint organic cherry tomatoes

Garnish: 4 tablespoons toasted chopped pecans,
¼ cup grated sheep's milk pecorino romano or
Parmesan Cheese Substitute (page 152), twist of
pepper, extra-virgin olive oil

In a large skillet, heat 2 tablespoons of sesame oil. Add the onion, garlic, and chili flakes and sauté all until the onion is caramelized. Then add the broccoli rabe to the skillet with the 2 tablespoons of water. Cover and cook the rabe until tender but still bright green. When done, immediately remove to a warm platter.

In the same skillet add the remaining 2 tablespoons of sesame oil and cook the cherry tomatoes, stirring occasionally, until the skins split.

To finish the dish, spoon the tomatoes on top of the broccoli rabe and sprinkle with the chopped pecans, cheese, and a twist of pepper. Drizzle with a little olive oil for extra glisten.

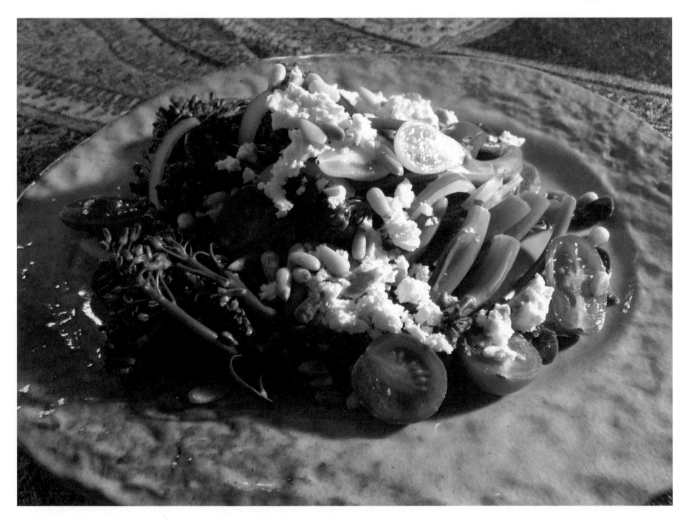

Asian Cauliflower "Fried Rice" with Egg Omelet

SERVES 6 GENEROUSLY

This dish can be an entrée instead of a side dish simply by adding leftover cooked seafood or meat. It's a great way to make a fast and tasty meal for the family.

The Cauliflower "Fried Rice"

1 large head cauliflower

3 to 4 tablespoons cold-pressed sesame oil or coconut oil

1 small onion, finely diced

4 ounces (or more) sliced shiitake mushrooms, tough stems removed

2 to 3 tablespoons freshly grated ginger

pinch of sea salt and freshly ground pepper, to taste

2 tablespoons Coconut Secret Raw Coconut Aminos

2 tablespoons fresh lime juice, rice wine vinegar, or coconut vinegar

2 tablespoons *each* chopped cilantro, mint, and basil leaves

Garnish: splash of Red Boat Fish Sauce*

The Egg Omelet

3 pastured eggs

1 tablespoon minced scallion, white and green parts

pinch of sea salt

1 tablespoon cold-pressed sesame oil or coconut oil

For the cauliflower fried rice: In a food processor, pulse the cauliflower until it resembles grains of rice.

In a large sauté pan, heat the sesame oil until medium hot. When the pan is hot, add the finely diced onion and sauté until translucent. Add the shitake mushrooms

---

*The primary ingredient in Red Boat is wild-caught black anchovy from the crystal-clear waters of the Phu Quoc island archipelago off the coast of Vietnam.

and stir-fry the mixture until the mushrooms are browned. Add the ginger and mix again, then add the cauliflower rice. Season with salt and pepper. Cover the pan and cook mixture for about 5 minutes, then add the coconut aminos, lime juice or vinegar, and herbs. Stir well and remove from heat.

For the omelet: Whisk the eggs in a bowl, then add the minced scallion and salt. In a very large sauté pan, heat the sesame oil to medium hot. Pour the eggs into the hot pan and fry the omelet very thin. When cooked on one side use a wide spatula to flip it over. Remove from pan, cool, and slice into thin strips. The omelet is now ready to add to the cauliflower rice.

To serve: Fold the egg omelet into the cauliflower rice. If you are using leftover seafood or meat in the dish, warm first, and then fold it in. Garnish with fish sauce. Serve while hot.

Haricots Verts Niçoise

SERVES 6

I love these delicate French green beans. This is a classic preparation served at room temperature, so it's perfect for a picnic or barbecue. The haricots verts make a fine accompaniment to a simply prepared chicken or fish.

1 tablespoon sea salt
1 pound haricots verts or any young garden bean
1 tablespoon extra-virgin olive oil
1 pint organic cherry tomatoes, halved
½ cup pitted Niçoise olives
Garnish: ¼ cup toasted pine nuts

Bring a large pot of salted water (enough to cover the beans) to a boil. Blanch the beans in the salted water for 2–3 minutes, then drop them into ice water to stop the cooking. The beans should be al dente and bright green. Drain and set aside.

Just before serving, toss the beans in a large bowl with the olive oil, tomatoes, and Niçoise olives. Arrange the beans on individual salad plates or put them in a pretty bowl and sprinkle with the toasted pine nuts.

Oregano Pesto Vegetables

SERVES 6

The oregano in the pesto gives it a complex flavor. For this dish,
use whatever vegetables you fancy. I make a suggestion of what you can use here.
Use any leftover pesto vegetables in your breakfast eggs.

The Oregano Pesto

- 6 to 8 large cloves garlic
- 2 large bunches basil leaves, about 4 cups
- 1 small bunch oregano leaves, about 1 cup
- ½ cup pine nuts or walnuts
- juice of ½ lemon
- ⅔ cup grated pecorino romano or Parmesan Cheese
  Substitute (page 152)
- 1 cup extra-virgin olive oil
- sea salt and a twist of pepper, to taste

The Vegetables

- 1 bunch kale, trimmed of stems
- 2 pounds asparagus, broccolini, summer squash, or
  cauliflower, or a combination
- 1 onion, halved and sliced
- 2 tablespoons cold-pressed sesame oil
- 1 red, yellow, or orange bell pepper
- Garnish: grated pecorino romano cheese or Parmesan
  Cheese Substitute (page 152)
- 1 cup organic cherry tomatoes, halved

For the pesto: In a food processor, combine the garlic, basil, oregano, pine nuts, lemon juice, and the cheese. With the processor running, slowly pour in the olive oil until the mixture is very smooth, adding more oil if necessary. Season to taste with the salt and pepper. Remove the pesto to a bowl, cover, and set aside while preparing the vegetables.

For the vegetables: Wash and prepare the vegetables by removing stems from kale, snapping the tough ends off the asparagus, trimming the ends off the broccolini stems, and cutting the squash and cauliflower into bite-size pieces.

In a large sauté pan, over medium heat, cook the onion in the sesame oil until golden brown. Add the remaining vegetables (except the tomatoes) and cover. Cook for a few minutes until just done. The vegetables should still be vibrant in color. Remove the cover and stir in the pesto, coating the vegetables thoroughly.

To serve: Turn the vegetables out onto a large platter and surround with the cherry tomatoes. For garnish sprinkle more cheese on top.

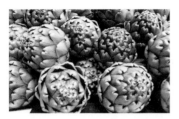

California Steamed Artichokes

FOR ANY NUMBER OF PEOPLE

My parents moved from Minnesota to the San Joaquin Valley in 1952 when I was six years old. When I started the first grade in Turlock, California, I went to my friend's house so we could walk together to school. My first introduction to artichokes was watching my friend and her family eating artichokes for breakfast. I have loved them ever since. In California, the large green globe artichokes come from Monterey County, particularly the town of Castroville, the self-proclaimed Artichoke Capitol of the World.

1 artichoke per person, or half if
   they're extra large
melted butter and lemon juice, for dipping

First, use a serrated knife to cut away the top of the artichoke about a third of the way between the tip and the base. Cut the stem from the bottom of the artichoke. I usually peel off a few of the tough outer leaves as well.

Bring water to a boil in a steamer and steam the artichokes until they are fork tender. Remove to a plate and place upside down to drain.

To serve, give each person their own artichoke on a salad plate. Give each individual a small bowl of melted butter and lemon juice. Homemade Mayonnaise (page 123), Garlic Aioli (page 152), or Bagna Cauda (page 87) are fabulous as well.

To eat an artichoke, peel off each leaf, dip the soft end of the leaf (where it attaches to the globe) in butter, and then scrape the tender part off with your teeth. This can be a very messy, drippy, eating fest; if you're a fastidious eater, artichokes probably are not for you. After you've eaten the leaves, scoop out the choke with a spoon and eat the creamy artichoke heart. Fantastic!

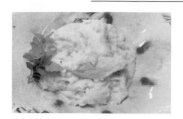

Cauliflower "Mashed Potatoes"

SERVES 4

I kid you not. I have fooled many people into thinking this dish was real mashed potatoes—even people who said they didn't like cauliflower. Mashed cauliflower is your alternative to starchy mashed potatoes, and it's just as satisfying. Serve them with any meat or fish that you'd normally serve with mashed potatoes, like roast chicken or meat loaf.

1½ to 2 pounds organic cauliflower, trimmed and cut into small pieces (one very large head or two small heads)

2 to 3 tablespoons pastured butter or ghee

3 to 4 tablespoons pastured cream or goat's milk, for consistency

2 to 3 ounces goat cheese

sea salt and freshly ground pepper, to taste

Place the cauliflower in a steamer and cook until tender. Transfer the steamed cauliflower to a food processor and pulse. Add the butter or ghee and a few tablespoons of cream and process the mixture until smooth. If you are using the goat cheese, add it with the cream and ghee. Add the salt and pepper to taste.

Oven-Roasted Asparagus

SERVES 4 AS A SIDE DISH

Spring asparagus is surely one of the great pleasures of life. Roasting adds a special flavor to asparagus.

The Basting Sauce

½ cup, very fruity extra-virgin olive oil

3 teaspoons minced garlic

¼ cup balsamic vinegar

The Asparagus

approximately 2 bunches fresh asparagus (3 to 4 spears per person)

Garnish: sea salt and freshly ground pepper, ½ cup
 grated sheep's milk pecorino romano or Parmesan
 Cheese Substitute (page 152)

Preheat the oven to 400 degrees.

For the basting sauce: In a bowl whisk together the basting ingredients.

For the asparagus: Snap off the ends of the asparagus spears, then place the asparagus in a large glass rectangular baking dish. Coat them thoroughly with half of the basting sauce. Arrange the asparagus on a stainless steel sheet pan and roast in the oven, turning them often, until they become bright green (6–9 minutes).

Remove the asparagus from the oven and coat the spears with the remaining half of the basting sauce, the grated cheese, salt, and pepper. At this point you can broil the asparagus for an additional minute.

To serve: Divide the asparagus onto four dinner plates or place on a large platter. Grate more cheese on top, if desired.

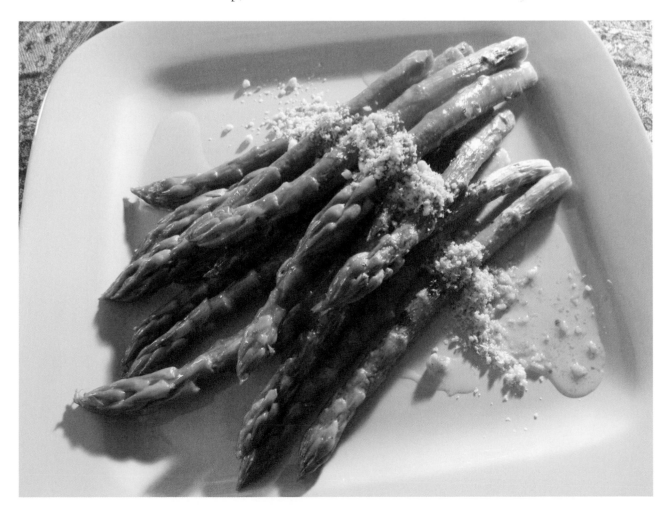

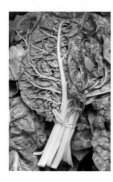

Sautéed Greens

SERVES 6

*I eat sautéed kale or chard a couple times a week. With the greens
I cook onions, plenty of garlic, and colorful bell peppers to add
flavor and color. This recipe is a very tasty way to
get your family to eat their greens.*

The Vegetables

  2 large bunches organic kale, Swiss chard, mustard
    greens, or spinach. You can mix them.
  2 tablespoons cold-pressed sesame oil
  1 medium yellow onion, thinly sliced
  6 cloves garlic, minced
  1 red bell pepper, seeded and thinly sliced
  ½ teaspoon sea salt and a twist of pepper
  2 tablespoons water

The Dressing

  juice of ½ lemon or 1 tablespoon balsamic vinegar
  2 tablespoons extra-virgin olive oil
  ¼ teaspoon red pepper flakes
  Garnish: grated sheep's milk pecorino romano or
    Parmesan Cheese Substitute (page 152)

For the vegetables: Wash greens and remove the leaves from the stems. You will cook the leaves only. In a large sauté skillet heat the oil and sauté the onion until nicely browned and crispy. Then add the garlic, sliced red pepper, and the greens. Season with the salt and pepper, and thoroughly toss all the ingredients. Add 2 tablespoons of water to the skillet and cover, letting the vegetables cook until just wilted but still bright green. You don't want to overcook the greens. Remove from heat.

   For the dressing: Whisk the ingredients together in a small bowl.

   To serve: Pour the dressing over the greens and toss like a salad. Turn them out onto a warm platter and garnish with the cheese.

Delicious Braised Cabbage

SERVES 6 TO 8

If you're a fan of braised cabbage, then you'll love this rendition. It will make a wonderful accompaniment to ham or roast loin of pork.

1 medium green cabbage (about 2 pounds), trimmed
   of outer leaves and core
1 yellow onion, sliced
1 large red bell pepper, stem removed, seeded, and
   sliced
¼ cup chicken stock or vegetable stock, recipes in
   soup section
¼ cup cold-pressed sesame oil (for a variation use
   hot rendered duck or bacon fat)
sea salt and freshly ground pepper, to taste
¼ teaspoon red pepper flakes, or to taste
2 teaspoons Coconut Secret Raw Coconut Vinegar,
   rice vinegar, or aged balsamic vinegar
Garnish: Maldon salt

Preheat the oven to 325 degrees. Lightly oil a 9 × 13-inch glass baking dish. Cut the trimmed cabbage into eight wedges. Arrange the wedges in a single layer in the dish. Cover the cabbage with the sliced onions and peppers. Mix together the stock and sesame oil or duck fat, and pour the mixture over the cabbage and onions. Season the top of the dish with the salt, pepper, and red pepper flakes.

Cover the dish with foil and place in the oven, braising for about two hours until the cabbage is tender. After one hour of cooking time, use a wide spatula to gently turn over the cabbage wedges. Continue cooking for another hour and then remove the cabbage from the oven. Increase the oven temperature to 400 degrees.

Sprinkle your choice of vinegar evenly over the cabbage and return the dish to the oven for another 15 minutes or so, until the cabbage begins to brown. Remove from the oven and sprinkle the cabbage with a little Maldon salt for sparkle, if desired.

Zucchini Noodles

SERVES 4 TO 6

Use zucchini noodles in place of traditional noodles with a rich tomato sauce or basil pesto. It is also wonderful with butter and grated cheese or Parmesan Cheese Substitute (page 152). The kids will love zucchini noodles, I guarantee.

1 teaspoon, or more, sea salt for lightly salted water
8 to 12 organic zucchini (more if desired)
pinch of sea salt and a twist of pepper

Bring a large pot of salted water (enough to cover the zucchini) to a boil.

First cut off both ends of the zucchini. Then, using a mandolin, if you have one, carefully slice the zucchini lengthwise from one end to the other. You can also lay the zucchini flat on a cutting board and cut the slices with a very sharp knife, about ¼-inch thick. A rustic look to the zucchini is fine. When you come to the tough seeded part of the zucchini, discard it. Use additional zucchini if you have to.

Add the zucchini slices to the boiling water and cook them quickly, 1–2 minutes. Remove the slices from the pot and plunge into ice water to stop the cooking. Now drain and remove the zucchini to a large bowl. Season with salt and pepper.

To serve, reheat the zucchini noodles and finish the preparation in whatever way you choose.

Italian-Style Peppers with Capers

SERVES 4

*I love colorful peppers. This is a simple, rustic side dish that can be
served with grilled fish, chicken, lamb kebobs, or flank steak.*

4 tablespoons cold-pressed sesame oil

2 large sweet onions, thinly sliced

2 yellow or orange bell peppers, thinly sliced

2 red bell peppers, thinly sliced

3 ripe organic tomatoes, peeled and chopped, or 4
   Muir Glen organic plum tomatoes

1 tablespoon red wine or balsamic vinegar

2 tablespoons extra-virgin olive oil

¼ cup salt-cured capers or regular capers, rinsed

In a large saucepan over medium heat, warm the sesame oil. Add the onions and
sauté until golden brown, 6–8 minutes. Add the peppers and cook 4–5 minutes, until
the liquid has evaporated and the peppers are soft. Add the tomatoes and continue
cooking for another 2–3 minutes, but do not let the tomatoes break down. They
should still be chunky.

Remove the mixture from the heat and add the vinegar, olive oil, and capers. Toss
the mixture well. Serve the peppers at room temperature.

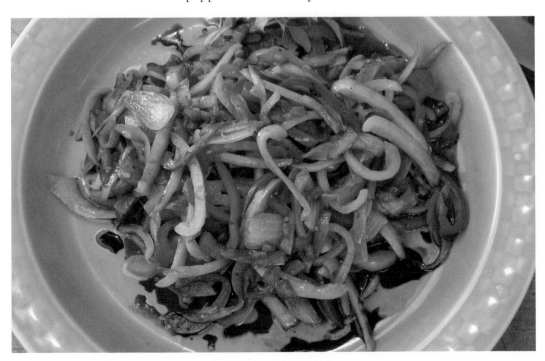

Roasted Winter Vegetables

SERVES 6

Winter vegetables make a very heartwarming dish when the weather is cold.
Serve the roasted vegetables with Bagna Cauda (page 87)
or Garlic Aioli (page 152).

1 large head cauliflower

1 large acorn squash, seeded and peeled

½ pound broccoli florets

6 small fennel bulbs

1 pound very fresh asparagus

4 tablespoons cold-pressed sesame oil

Garnish: 1 head Belgian endive and 1 head radicchio
  or Traviso (red leaf chicory), Maldon sea salt,
  freshly ground pepper

Bring a large pot of water to a boil, and preheat the oven to 400 degrees.

Trim the cauliflower into small pieces, removing the core. Halve the acorn squash and scoop out the seeds. With a sharp knife, remove the peel and then cut the squash into pieces about 1-inch long and ¼-inch wide. Trim the broccoli into small florets. Cut the fennel into thin wedges, keeping the root end intact. Snap the tough ends off the asparagus.

In the boiling water, blanch the vegetables, one at a time, beginning with the cauliflower, then the fennel, squash, asparagus, and broccoli. Bring the water to a boil each time you add another vegetable. Cook vegetables until just done but still crisp. Lift the vegetables out of the pot with a slotted spoon or tongs and plunge into ice water to stop the cooking. Remove the vegetables to a waiting platter.

When all the vegetables have been blanched, heat the sesame oil in a large sauté pan. Add the cooked and drained vegetables, stirring gently, and heating the vegetables thoroughly. At this point you can turn the vegetables out onto a stainless steel sheet pan and roast them in the oven until lightly browned.

To serve, arrange the Belgian endive and radicchio leaves attractively on six salad plates. Then place the warmed vegetables on top. Sprinkle the vegetables with a little Maldon salt and give them a twist of pepper. Put small bowls of aioli or bagna cauda on the table so everyone can help themselves.

Spaghetti Squash Gratin

SERVES 6

Spaghetti squash is fun. This gratin makes a good Thanksgiving side dish as a replacement for overly sweet baked yams with marshmallows. One day I had some ground nuts left from baking a tart, and I sprinkled them on top of the gratin before baking. The nuts really dressed it up.

The Squash

    2 pounds spaghetti squash, halved lengthwise, cut
        side brushed with sesame oil

The Gratin Topping

    2 tablespoons ghee or cold-pressed sesame oil

    2 cups thinly sliced onions

    3 to 4 cloves garlic, minced

    2 cups chicken stock or vegetable stock (recipes in
        soup section)

    sea salt and freshly ground pepper, to taste

    1 tablespoon fresh thyme, chopped

    ½ cup pastured cream or coconut cream

    1 cup grated sheep's milk manchego, Parmesan
        Cheese Substitute (page 152), or ground nuts

    Garnish: 2 tablespoons minced parsley

Preheat the oven to 350 degrees.

For the squash: Place the squash, cut side down, in a 9 × 13-inch glass baking dish. Bake the squash for about 40 minutes, or until fork tender. Remove from the oven, scoop out the seeds, and then scoop the pulp into an oiled gratin dish. Spread the squash evenly in the dish.

Turn the oven to broil.

For the gratin topping: In a large skillet, sauté the onions and garlic in the ghee 6–8 minutes, until light brown. Add the stock, salt, pepper, and thyme and bring the mixture to a boil. Pour the onion broth over the squash. Bake the gratin for 30 minutes. Remove from oven and drizzle the cream and cheese over the top of the dish. Return to the oven and bake until the top is brown and bubbly.

When serving, garnish the gratin with the minced parsley.

Chili Rellenos with Fresh Herb Salsa

SERVES 6

Chili rellenos can be a sensational main entrée or side dish. The result is well worth the effort of blistering and peeling the chilies. I served these as a first course for Christmas dinner in Santa Fe, followed by roast turkey with Mexican mole. I cannot imagine a more special Christmas dinner. Serve the chili rellenos with salad greens, avocados, radishes, oranges, and a citrus vinaigrette. If you have leftover rellenos, add them into your breakfast eggs.

The Chilies

12 anaheim chilies or poblano chilies (I like the
   meaty poblano chilies)

The Filling

8 ounces goat cheese, softened

2 cloves garlic, minced

2 tablespoons shallots, minced

8 ounces grated sheep's milk manchego

1 ripe organic tomato, diced

¼ cup cilantro leaves, chopped

½ cup basil leaves, julienned

sea salt and a twist of pepper, to taste

The Fresh Herb Salsa

2 shallots, finely minced

½ cup Champagne vinegar

¾ cup extra-virgin olive oil

3 ripe organic tomatoes, peeled, seeded, and diced

1 tablespoon each of fresh thyme, oregano, and
   flat-leaf parsley

The Chili Coating Mixture

¼ teaspoon sea salt and a twist of pepper

1 egg

2 tablespoons pastured cream or goat's milk

2 cups finely ground almonds for coating

cold-pressed sesame oil for frying

For the chilies: Prepare the chilies by blistering the skins over the fire on your gas burner or under the broiler in the oven. Keep turning the chilies so they blister evenly. Then place them in a brown paper bag to steam. When cool enough, peel off the skins under running water or in a bowl of water. Use gloves for this; you don't want to wipe your eyes and get chili seed oil in them.

Slice open the chilies lengthwise and remove the seeds, being careful not to tear the chilies. If you do happen to tear them, you can press them together again when you put the filling inside.

For the filling: In a bowl combine the goat cheese, garlic, shallots, manchego, tomato, cilantro, basil, sea salt, and pepper. Gently stuff the filling into the chilies and secure them with a toothpick. Set the chilies aside.

For the fresh herb salsa: In a bowl whisk together the ingredients. Set aside.

For the chili coating: In another bowl, beat the egg and cream (or goat's milk) together with the salt and pepper and pour this mixture into a pie pan. Place the ground nuts on a plate. While the sesame oil is heating in a large skillet, roll each chili in the egg-and-cream mixture, then in the ground almonds. Fry the chilies until they are golden brown all around. Place them in a shallow baking dish in a warm oven until ready to serve.

To serve: Spoon the salsa over the rellenos.

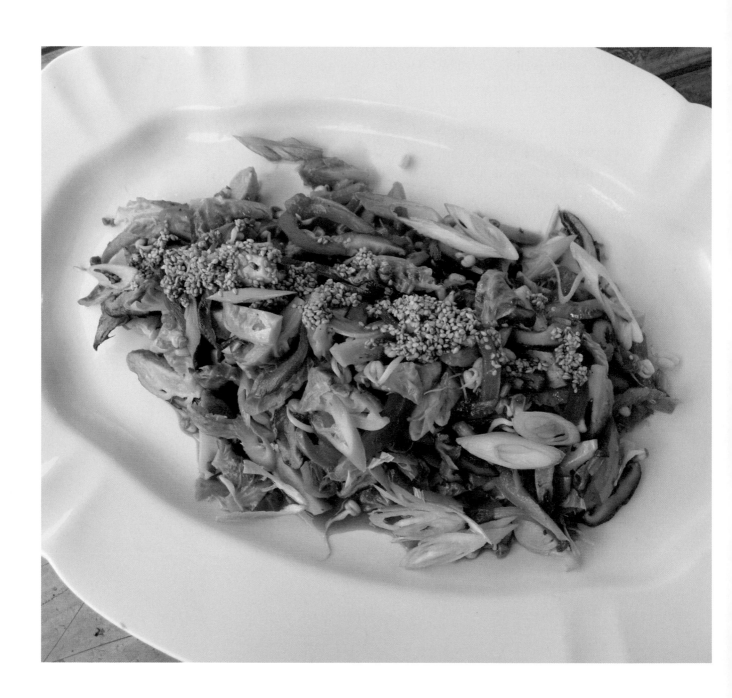

Japanese Brussels Sprouts
with Shiitake Mushrooms

SERVES 6

I love shiitake mushrooms and Brussels sprouts when they are prepared in an interesting way. This hearty dish is full of flavor. If your family likes Asian food, they will love this version of Brussels sprouts.

4 tablespoons cold-pressed sesame oil

½ small onion, sliced

1 red bell pepper, seeded and very thinly sliced

1½ pounds Brussels sprouts, trimmed and halved

6 ounces fresh shiitake mushrooms, stems removed
    and sliced, approximately 1 cup

1 tablespoon minced garlic

½ cup chicken or vegetable stock (pages 102–3)

2 tablespoons rice wine vinegar

2 tablespoons mirin (Japanese rice cooking wine),
    optional

2 tablespoons Coconut Secret Raw Coconut Aminos*

2 cups mung bean sprouts, rinsed

Garnish: 2 scallions, thinly sliced on the diagonal;
    toasted sesame seeds

Heat the sesame oil in a large sauté pan or wok, and cook the onion, bell pepper, and Brussels sprouts about 3 minutes. Add the sliced shiitakes and cook the mixture another 3 minutes. The Brussels sprouts should be bright green. Add the minced garlic, and cook an additional 2 minutes. Then add the stock and continue cooking until the liquid is almost evaporated.

Add the rice wine vinegar, mirin, and coconut aminos to the vegetable mixture and then toss in the mung bean sprouts and mix well.

To serve, immediately turn the vegetables out onto a platter and garnish with the scallions and toasted sesame seeds.

---

*Coconut Aminos replaces tamari for those who cannot consume foods containing gluten or soy.

Broccoli, Sicilian Style

SERVES 8

This is a quick and unusual broccoli recipe that's great for a party or for the holidays.

2 pounds broccoli, cut into small florets (you can use
 broccolini)
pinch of sea salt and a twist of pepper
4 tablespoons cold-pressed sesame oil
3 medium onions, thinly sliced
½ cup Zinfandel (optional), or use chicken or
 vegetable stock
2 tablespoons red wine vinegar
1 tablespoon organic tomato paste
½ teaspoon fresh oregano
¼ teaspoon red chili flakes
4 cloves garlic, thinly sliced
4 sprigs Italian (flat leaf) parsley
28 ounces (1 can) Muir Glen organic plum tomatoes,
 crushed, liquid reserved
⅓ cup pitted, oil-cured olives or Kalamata olives
¼ cup organic golden raisins, optional
⅓ cup toasted pine nuts
Garnish: grated sheep's milk pecorino romano or
 Parmesan Cheese Substitute (page 152)

Steam the broccoli in a vegetable steamer or in a small amount of water in a covered saucepan for about 6–8 minutes. Broccoli should be bright green. Transfer the broccoli to a large platter. Season it with salt and pepper. Cover and set aside in a slightly warm oven.

In a large, medium-hot skillet, heat the oil. Add the onions and cook until lightly browned. Add the wine or stock, vinegar, tomato paste, oregano, pepper flakes, garlic, and parsley and cook, stirring occasionally, until the mixture is reduced and thick, 4–5 minutes. Add the plum tomatoes with their liquid and bring the sauce to a boil. Lower the heat to medium low and simmer, uncovered, stirring occasionally, about 8–10 minutes. Add the olives and simmer the mixture about 10 minutes longer. Stir in the raisins.

To serve, spoon the sauce over the room-temperature broccoli and sprinkle the broccoli with toasted pine nuts. Pass the grated pecorino or Parmesan Cheese Substitute.

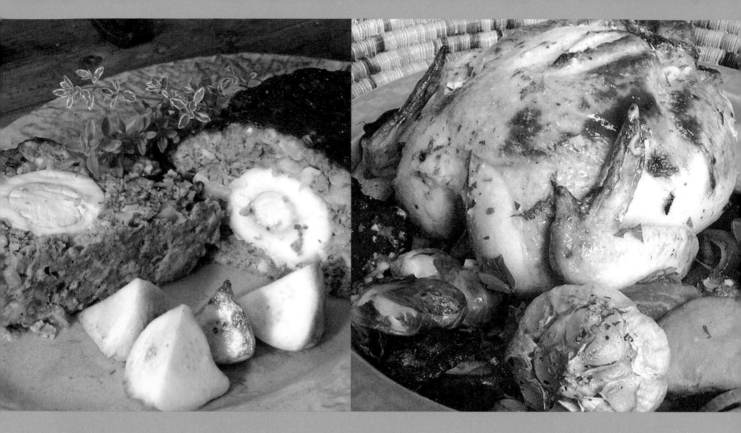

WHAT'S FOR DINNER?

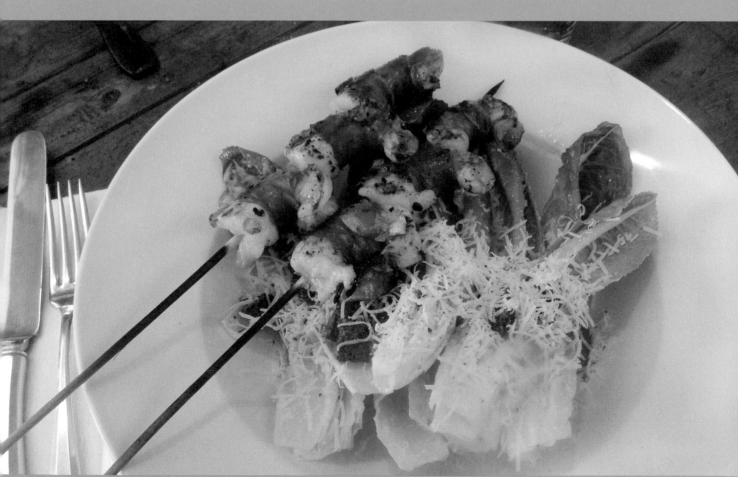

WILD-CAUGHT SEAFOOD

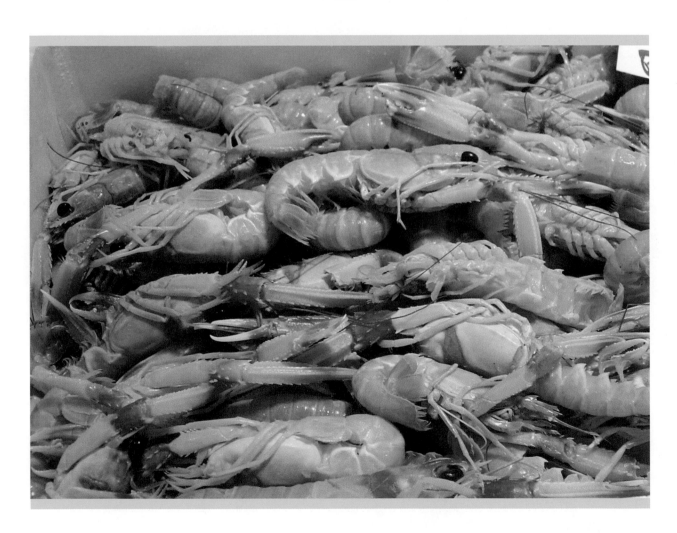

Pan-seared Salmon with Yogurt-Dill Sauce

SERVES 4

This is a classic dish that takes minutes to prepare. The whole-milk goat yogurt is as rich as sour cream. Serve the salmon with a great salad and your favorite grilled vegetables.

The Salmon

- 4 wild-caught salmon escallops, 3–4 ounces per person
- sea salt* and freshly ground pepper, to taste
- cold-pressed sesame oil
- 6 cups of fresh watercress and arugula, or other favorite greens
- extra-virgin olive oil for dressing the greens

The Yogurt-Dill Sauce

- 1 cup Capretta Rich and Creamy Goat Yogurt or Green Valley lactose-free sour cream
- 3 tablespoons Champagne vinegar
- 3 tablespoons whole-grain or Dijon mustard
- 6 tablespoons fresh dill, chopped
- 4 scallions, white and green parts, very finely minced

For the salmon: Place the salmon on a plate and sprinkle evenly with the salt and pepper.

In a large bowl toss the greens with some olive oil, making sure to coat the leaves well. Divide the greens among four dinner plates.

In a heavy-bottomed skillet heat the sesame oil to medium hot. Sear the salmon on each side for about one minute or a little longer. The salmon should remain nice and pink in the center.

For the yogurt-dill sauce: In a bowl mix together the yogurt, vinegar, mustard, dill, and scallions. Set the sauce aside.

To serve: Place the salmon on top of the greens. Drizzle the yogurt-dill sauce over the salmon.

---

*Celtic salt or Hawaiian pink salt is great for fish.

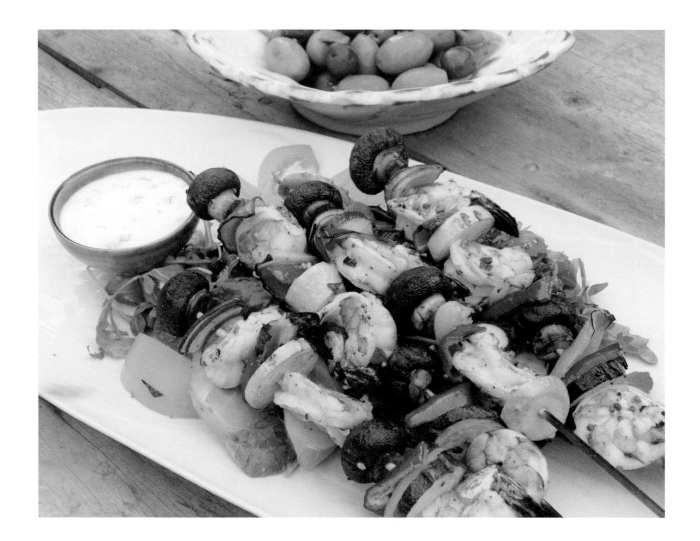

Grilled Prawn Kebabs with Chipotle, Cilantro & Lime Dipping Sauce

SERVES 4

The flavors of chipotle, cilantro, and lime are straight from Mexico.

Chipotle, Cilantro & Lime Dipping Sauce

¾ cup Capretta Rich and Creamy Goat Yogurt or
  thick coconut milk

1 teaspoon chipotle peppers,* minced

1 teaspoon chipotle adobo sauce

1 teaspoon cilantro leaves, finely chopped

½ teaspoon grated lime zest

1 tablespoon lime juice

1 teaspoon minced garlic

¼ teaspoon sea salt

The Kebabs

3 to 4 jumbo prawns per person

2 red bell peppers, cut into 1-inch pieces

1 red onion, cut into 1-inch pieces

8 large mushrooms

8 pieces summer squash, cut into 1-inch pieces

sesame oil for brushing skewers

sea salt, to taste

For the chipotle, cilantro & lime dipping sauce: In a bowl mix the sauce ingredients. Adjust the seasonings to taste. Cover and refrigerate for at least two hours.

For the kebabs: Alternate prawns, red bell pepper pieces, red onion, mushrooms, and squash on long, wooden skewers that have been soaked in water for an hour. Then brush the skewers with sesame oil and sprinkle with sea salt, to taste. Cook the kebabs on a hot grill or broil them for 2–3 minutes per side.

Serve the kebabs with small bowls of dipping sauce for each person.

---

*Chipotle peppers are available in small cans in the Mexican section of the grocery store.

Red Snapper Vera Cruz

SERVES 6

For a bright and festive dinner, this dish takes just minutes to make. Serve red snapper with a favorite vegetable. Try serving it with Cauliflower Rice (page 160) and a salad of greens, oranges, avocados, and Citrus Vinaigrette (page 121). Halibut is a good alternative fish.

> 6 3-ounce pieces of Pacific red snapper fillet
> sea salt and freshly ground pepper, to taste
> 2 tablespoons ghee or cold-pressed sesame oil
> 1 large onion, seeded and thinly sliced
> ½ red bell pepper, thinly sliced
> 6 cloves garlic, minced
> 2 tablespoons jalapeños, seeded and chopped
> 4 organic Muir Glen or San Marzano plum tomatoes, chopped
> ¾ cup fish stock or ½ cup white wine and ¼ cup water
> juice of 1 lime
> ½ cup green olives, pitted and chopped (picholine olives or Lucques olives)
> 1 tablespoon fresh oregano
> 2 tablespoons pastured butter or goat butter
> Garnish: 2 tablespoons fresh parsley, chopped, and 3 limes cut into wedges

Season the snapper fillets with the salt and pepper. Set aside.

Heat the ghee in a large skillet over medium-high heat. Add the onion and cook, stirring occasionally, until golden, about 5–7 minutes. Add the red bell pepper, garlic, and jalapeño and cook 1 minute longer.

Add the tomatoes, fish stock, and lime juice and cook until the liquid is almost evaporated, 6–8 minutes. Stir in the olives and oregano. Add the snapper to the pan with the sauce and reduce the heat to medium. Cover and cook until the fish is opaque, about 5 minutes.

To serve, transfer the snapper to 6 dinner plates, leaving the sauce in the pan. With the sauce still in the pan, on high heat, add the butter and whisk until it coats a spoon. Then spoon the sauce over the fish. Sprinkle with the chopped parsley and garnish with the lime wedges.

Sautéed Sole
with Browned Butter & Capers

SERVES 2

Sole is always a favorite because of its delicacy. Fine accompaniments to the browned butter sauce would be creamed cauliflower and steamed Brussels sprouts.

The Fish

> 2 Pacific Rock Sole fillets, or Dover or Petrale sole,
>   about 3 ounces each
> sea salt and a twist of freshly ground pepper
> ¼ cup pastured cream
> ¼ cup almond flour
> 4 tablespoons ghee or cold-pressed sesame oil for
>   frying fish

The Browned Butter Sauce

> 4 tablespoons pastured butter
> juice of 1 lemon
> 2 teaspoons capers
> 2 tablespoons Italian (flat leaf) parsley, chopped
> pinch of sea salt and a twist of pepper

Place a large serving plate in the oven to warm at 200 degrees.

For the fish: Season the sole fillets with the salt and pepper and place them in a glass pie pan. Cover with the cream and set aside. Put the almond flour on a plate. Remove the fillets from the cream and dredge both sides in the flour.

In a large sauté pan, over medium heat, warm the ghee or sesame oil. Brown the fillets on both sides, carefully cooking the fish for about 2 minutes or longer. Transfer the sole immediately to the warmed plate.

To make the sauce: In the same sauté pan that you cooked the fish, over medium-high heat, add the butter and cook until it turns golden brown and has a nutty aroma. Immediately remove the pan from the heat and whisk in the lemon juice, capers, and parsley.

To serve: Quickly remove the sole from the oven and place the fillets on 2 dinner plates. Pour the browned butter sauce over the fish.

Salmon Niçoise with
Haricots Verts & Pastured Eggs
SERVES 8

For an easy summer supper this is a simple entrée that can be prepared in advance and assembled just before serving. The Lemon Oregano Dressing is a perfect match for the salmon. As an alternative to salmon, try Hawaiian tombo ahi (albacore tuna).

The Marinade

2 tablespoons extra-virgin olive oil

juice of 1 lemon

1 teaspoon minced fresh thyme

1 teaspoon lemon zest

½ cup finely minced scallions, white and green parts

¼ cup Italian (flat leaf) parsley, chopped

pinch of sea salt and freshly ground pepper

The Fish

1½ to 2 pounds Alaskan wild-caught salmon fillet, skin on

The Salad Accompaniments

1 pound steamed haricots verts or another young, tender garden bean

8 ounces your favorite salad greens: arugula, red oak leaf lettuce, watercress, or mesclun

8 hard-boiled eggs, peeled and cut into wedges

½ cup Niçoise olives, pitted

½ cup thinly sliced radishes

Garnish: avocado slices ($1/4$ avocado per person), sprigs of thyme, Maldon sea salt, and a twist of pepper

Lemon Oregano Dressing (page 121)

Preheat the oven to 400 degrees.

For the marinade: In a small bowl whisk together the olive oil, lemon juice, thyme, lemon zest, scallions, parsley, salt, and pepper. Set aside.

For the fish: Place the salmon, skin side down, in a large rectangular glass baking dish. Pour the marinade over the salmon and bake for 15–20 minutes, or until just done. Salmon should be slightly pink and moist in the center. Remove the salmon from the oven, and when cool enough gently remove the skin.

For the haricots verts: In a pot with a steamer basket, steam the haricots verts until crisp and bright green. Plunge into ice water to stop cooking.

To serve: Begin by tearing the salmon into 2-inch pieces with a fork. Place some of the salad greens on each dinner plate, arranging the hard-boiled egg wedges, radishes, and haricots verts artfully around the plate. Divide the salmon evenly over the greens and garnish with the Niçoise olives, avocado slices, and sprigs of fresh thyme. Spoon the dressing liberally over the salmon and the greens. For additional sparkle sprinkle the Maldon salt around the dish. Pass the pepper grinder.

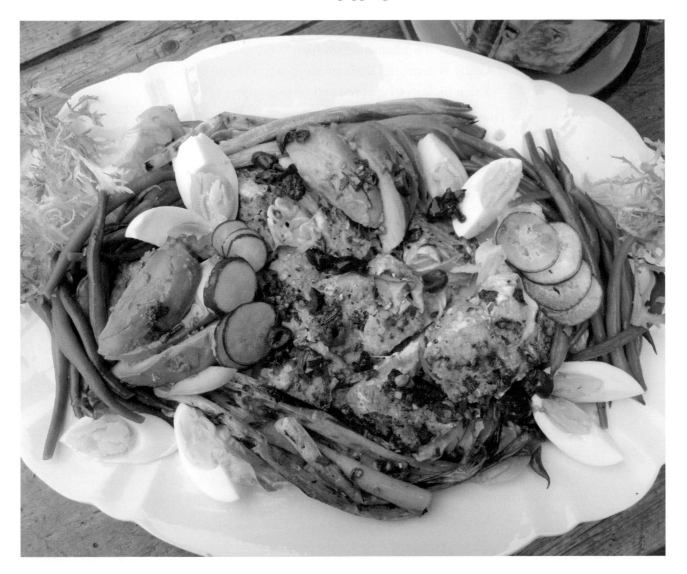

Hickory Grilled Salmon with Pistachio Sauce & Grilled Vegetables

This fabulous party dish was on our Best of Everything catering menus for years and was always a wedding favorite. Be sure to use wild-caught salmon. The combination of the pink salmon and the slightly green pistachio sauce is beautiful. For the grilled vegetables, we used asparagus, red onion wedges, eggplant, red bell peppers, cooked carrots, and prebaked sweet potato slices. We brushed the veggies generously with our special balsamic marinade. Everyone loved these vegetables.

The Salmon

1 very thick side of wild-caught Alaskan salmon*
   skin on (figure 3 ounces salmon per person)
sesame oil for brushing on fish
Celtic sea salt or Hawaiian pink salt, to taste
1 cup hickory chips, presoaked in water

The Pistachio Sauce

Enough for 12 generous servings of sauce.

1 cup freshly squeezed lemon juice
1 cup freshly squeezed orange juice
1 cup shelled unsalted pistachios
1 cup extra-virgin olive oil
½ teaspoon sea salt and a twist of pepper, to taste

The Grilled Vegetable Marinade

1 cup cold-pressed sesame oil
1 cup balsamic vinegar
3 to 4 shallots, finely minced
8 cloves garlic, finely minced
sea salt and freshly ground pepper, to taste

---

*Alaskan wild salmon is considered a "best choice" and is certified sustainable. Fishery management is especially important for salmon as these fish require both freshwater and ocean habitats to survive and reproduce.

The Grilled Vegetables

The quantity of vegetables used is determined by the number of guests. I leave that up to the cook to determine.

prebaked sweet potatoes, sliced about 1 inch thick (optional)

asparagus, tough ends removed

red onion wedges

eggplant slices, cut about 1-inch thick

large mushrooms

red bell pepper, seeded and cut into large chunks

zucchini, sliced down the middle, lengthwise

vine-ripened tomatoes, halved

whole scallions

For the salmon: Brush the salmon with sesame oil and then sprinkle lightly with the sea salt. Place the salmon, skin side down, on an oiled sheet of aluminum foil to place later on the grill.

For the pistachio sauce: In a blender add the lemon juice, orange juice, and pistachios and blend until very smooth. With the blender still running, slowly add the olive oil until the sauce thickens. The consistency of the sauce should be pourable, so adjust with more of the juices to suite your taste. Season with the salt and pepper. Cover the sauce and set aside.

For the grill: To prepare the grill, place the charcoal at one side of the grill and light it. When the charcoal has burned down to a moderately hot heat, drain the water off the hickory chips and add them on top of the coals. Place the salmon on the grill opposite the coals.

Cover the grill, allowing just enough air flow to maintain the heat. Grill the fish indirectly until the juices begin to flow and the salmon exhibits some resistance to the touch about 15–20 minutes. The finished salmon will be a mahogany color.

Remove the fish to a large oval platter and garnish with the pistachio sauce.

For the marinade and vegetables: Mix the marinade ingredients in a bowl. Set aside while you prep the vegetables. After preparing the vegetables, arrange them on a large sheet pan and brush liberally with the marinade.

Light the grill and bring the temperature to medium-hot. Place the vegetables on the grill (you may have to grill them in batches). As you grill the vegetables keep brushing on more marinade, turning the vegetables as they cook. When done, remove vegetables to a large platter and brush with the marinade once more for extra sheen.

Mahi-mahi Fish Tacos
with Butter Lettuce "Tortillas"

SERVES 6

I could eat fish tacos almost every day. Everyone loves them, and they make a very economical and simple meal. The whole family can participate in the preparation. The tacos are great served with the Mexican Cole Slaw with Chipotle-Lime Dressing (page 150). Yummy!

The Fish

3 ounces per person Pacific mahi-mahi or farm-raised tilapia*
sea salt and a twist of pepper, to taste

Yogurt-Lime Dressing

1 pint Capretta Rich and Creamy Goat Yogurt or
   lactose-free sour cream
3 tablespoons lime juice
2 cloves garlic, minced
several drops of bottled chipotle hot sauce, optional
Garnish: guacamole (recipe below), 1 cup grated sheep's milk
   manchego or raw cheddar or jack cheese

Guacamole

2 to 3 large, ripe avocados, peeled, pitted, and
   roughly chopped
1 or 2 scallions, white and green parts, minced
lime juice, to taste
1 to 2 cloves garlic, minced, optional
1 jalapeño, seeded and minced
pinch of sea salt and a twist of pepper, to taste

The Toppings

12 large leaves of red leaf butter lettuce
5 large, ripe tomatoes, peeled, seeded, and chopped
1 large red onion, very thinly sliced
leaves from 1 bunch of cilantro

---

*I use the delicious frozen wild-caught mahi-mahi from Trader Joe's. The Monterey Aquarium's Seafood Watch Best Choice is Pacific mahi-mahi, and U.S.-farmed tilapia is also rated well.

2 poblano chilies, charred, peeled, seeded, and
   chopped, optional
5 jalapeños, seeds removed and chopped
2 cups red and green cabbage, shredded (eliminate
   the cabbage if making the cole slaw)

For the fish: Add sea salt and pepper to the fish and then broil or grill to your taste. When done, tear the fish into pieces, cover, and keep warm.

For the yogurt-lime dressing: In a bowl mix together the ingredients for the dressing. Set aside.

For the guacamole: In a small bowl mash the avocados with a fork, leaving them somewhat chunky. In another small bowl place the scallions and the lime juice and let sit for a minute. Combine avocados, scallion mixture, and garlic and then add the jalapeno and salt and pepper. Adjust flavors to suite your taste.

To serve: In separate bowls, place the torn fish, tomatoes, red onion slices, cilantro leaves, grilled poblano chilies, jalapeños, shredded cabbage, guacamole, and lime wedges. Place the lettuce leaves on a plate. Let each person make his or her own taco.

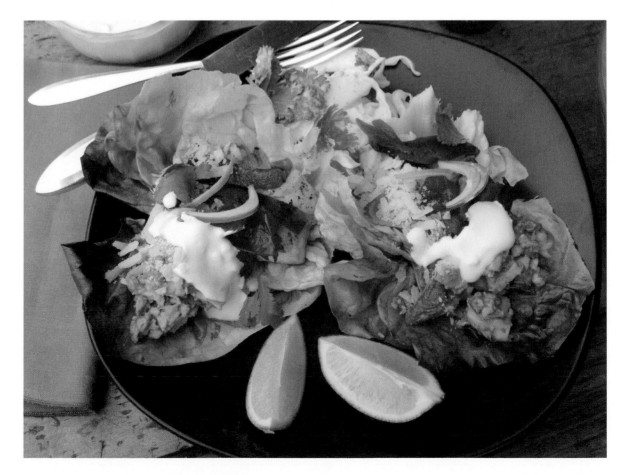

Sweet-and-Sour Hawaiian Snapper

SERVES 4

Hawaiian snapper is very tasty and absorbs flavors well. Perfect for company, this chilled dish is made the day before it is served to give the snapper time to marinate in the sauce. Serve the fish with a summer salad and grilled asparagus.

The Fish

4 3-ounce pieces Hawaiian snapper fillets*

Celtic sea salt or Hawaiian pink salt, to taste

freshly ground pepper, to taste

¼ cup coconut flour or almond flour (both are gluten-free)

¾ cup coconut oil or cold-pressed sesame oil

Garnish: celery ribbons (1 celery stalk, 6 inches in length, sliced into paper-thin ribbons), juice of ½ lemon, 2 tablespoons extra-virgin olive oil

The Marinade

¼ cup coconut oil or cold-pressed sesame oil

1 small red onion, halved and thinly sliced

¼ cup organic golden raisins

¼ cup pine nuts

Stevita brand stevia, to taste (add sparingly if you desire additional sweetness to the sauce)

¾ cup red wine vinegar

3 tablespoons chives or scallions, very finely diced

For the fish: Season the snapper with the salt and pepper and then dust the fish with the coconut flour on both sides.

In a heavy-bottomed skillet, heat the oil to medium hot and fry the fish on both sides until nicely browned, about 4–6 minutes. Remove the fish and drain on paper towels.

---

*Hawaiian snapper is a "good" seafood choice.

For the marinade: Wipe out the skillet with a paper towel and, over medium heat, heat the oil. Add the onion and cook until translucent, about 10 minutes. Add the raisins, pine nuts, stevia, vinegar, and chives and bring the mixture to a boil. Cook for 5–6 minutes, remove from heat and cool.

In a glass bowl, layer the snapper pieces and the marinade, ending with the marinade on top. Press plastic wrap on top of the dish to make it airtight. Refrigerate for approximately 24 hours. Remove from the refrigerator 1 hour before serving.

To serve: Just before serving, toss the celery ribbons in a bowl with the lemon juice and olive oil and toss well. Season ever so slightly with salt and pepper.

To serve, place the snapper pieces in the center of 4 salad plates and spoon the marinade evenly over the fish. Garnish each plate with a mound of celery ribbons.

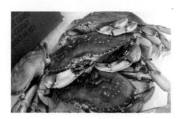

Mardi Gras
Crab Cakes
with Creole Remoulade

SERVES 4

I love crab cakes. I test a restaurant by how good their crab cakes are. Crab cakes require impeccably fresh crab. Dungeness crabs are caught all along the Pacific coast—from Alaska to Baja—from November to June. Crab cakes make a lovely brunch dish or a simple Sunday night supper. The Creole Remoulade is not your typical seafood sauce. It is very complex and works perfectly with the crab cakes or as a seafood cocktail sauce. You can also use it as a party dip for shrimp.

The Crab Cakes

- 1 pound Dungeness crab* meat
- ¼ cup Homemade Mayonnaise (page 123)
- 1 bunch scallions, white and green parts, minced
- ¼ cup red bell pepper, finely chopped
- 1 egg, beaten
- 1 teaspoon lemon juice
- ½ cup almond meal (finely ground almonds)
- dash of Tabasco
- pinch of sea salt and a twist of pepper
- more almond meal for coating the crab cakes, about ½ cup
- ¼ cup sesame oil for frying

The Creole Remoulade
Make at least 6 hours in advance.

- juice of 1 lemon
- peel of 1 organic lemon
- 1 egg
- ⅓ cup Natural Value Organic Horseradish Mustard[†]
- 1 teaspoon sea salt
- 1 teaspoon paprika

---

*Dungeness crabs are a "good," sustainable seafood choice

[†]Most prepared horseradish products contain gluten. Natural Value Organic Horseradish Mustard lists organic horseradish as an ingredient. You can always grate fresh horseradish if you prefer.

1 cup extra virgin olive oil

¼ cup Champagne vinegar

2 cloves garlic, minced

1 tablespoon flat-leaf parsley, minced

1 shallot, minced

4 tablespoons minced celery leaf

2 teaspoons aged balsamic vinegar*

1 bay leaf

For the crab cakes: If the crab meat has been frozen, squeeze out the excess water before proceeding with the recipe.

In a bowl combine all the ingredients—except the sesame oil. Mix until well blended, but do not break the large pieces of crab meat. Shape the mixture into 4 patties that are approximately 3 inches in diameter. If the mixture does not hold together, add a little more almond meal.

Put the almond meal on a plate and coat the outside of the crab cakes on both sides. In a large skillet heat the oil on medium high. Fry the crab cakes on both sides to a light golden brown. Transfer to a paper towel–lined plate and keep warm until ready to serve.

For the Creole remoulade: Using a paring knife, trim peel off lemon, thinly, so there is no white part (pith). Juice the lemon. Set rind and juice aside.

In a small bowl, whisk together the egg, horseradish mustard, salt, and paprika. Gradually whisk in the oil until emulsified. Whisk in vinegar, lemon juice, garlic, parsley, shallot, celery leaf, and balsamic vinegar. Add the lemon rind and bay leaf and stir. Place the mixture in a jar and refrigerate for 6 hours or overnight, then remove the bay leaf and lemon rind.

To serve: Place the hot crab cakes on a salad plate and drape with the remoulade sauce. A nice accompaniment to the crab cakes would be a lightly dressed salad of mixed lettuces and a citrusy dressing.

---

*Balsamic vinegar replaces Worchestershire sauce, which lists wheat and soy in the ingredients.

Striped Sea Bass & Tangerines

SERVES 5

The delicious combination of sea bass and tangerines makes a bright and festive company entrée. Serve with the Savory Green Salad (page 124) and steamed haricots verts or oven-roasted asparagus. Make sure to leave enough time to marinate the sea bass before cooking.

The Marinade

zest of 2 tangerines

2 teaspoons fresh thyme leaves

1½ tablespoons Italian (flat leaf) parsley, chopped

The Fish

1 pound striped sea bass* fillets (about 3 ounces per person)

sea salt and freshly ground pepper, to taste

3 tangerines, peeled and divided into segments

2 tablespoons cold-pressed sesame oil

1½ cups fresh tangerine juice

4 tablespoons pastured butter or goat butter

Garnish: sprigs of thyme

In a bowl combine the zest, thyme, and parsley. Coat the fish fillets with the marinade mixture and refrigerate, covered, 4–5 hours. Bring the fish to room temperature about 20 minutes before cooking. Season with a little sea salt and pepper.

With a very sharp knife, remove the peeling from the tangerines, pith and all. Then slice between the membranes to release each individual segment. Place the segments in a bowl.

In a large sauté pan, over medium heat, add the sesame oil. Sauté the fish, skin side down, until the skin is crisp and light brown, about 3–4 minutes. Turn the fish and cook a few minutes until it is just done. Be careful not to overcook the fish.

---

*Sea bass farms in the United States are well managed, and the fish are raised in ponds or tanks.

Wipe out the pan and return it to the medium-high heat. Add the tangerine juice and bring to a boil. Reduce the juice by half and then whisk in the butter. Remove from heat and add the tangerine segments.

To serve, place a piece of bass on each dinner plate with the Savory Green Salad and vegetable of your choice. Spoon the sauce and the tangerine segments over the fish. Garnish with sprigs of thyme.

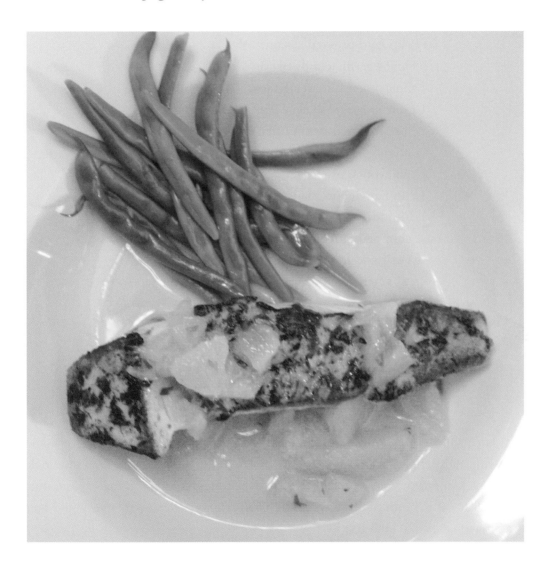

Cacciucco

SERVES 8 ABUNDANTLY

I had the best Tuscan seafood stew of my life in a restaurant in Florence, Italy, with my friend Sharon Dellamonica. After I ate the dish once, I went back to the restaurant and ate it again. The fish and shellfish were impeccably fresh. This is a special dish to be shared with friends and a good crisp white wine.

¼ cup cold-pressed sesame oil

6 cloves garlic, chopped

1 tablespoon Italian (flat leaf) parsley, chopped

1 tablespoon fresh sage leaves, chopped

½ teaspoon red pepper flakes

½ pound calamari, cleaned and cut into 1-inch pieces

1 tablespoon organic tomato paste

1 cup Sauvignon Blanc

1 14-ounce can Muir Glen organic plum tomatoes, chopped, juice reserved

sea salt and freshly ground pepper, to taste

2 cups fish stock or vegetable stock (recipes in soup section)

4 tablespoons pastured butter

1 pound red snapper cut into 2-inch pieces

1 pound large shrimp* with heads and shells

1 pound mussels[†]

Garnish: very fruity extra-virgin olive oil

In a large soup pot over medium heat, add the sesame oil, then the garlic, parsley, sage, and red pepper flakes. Cook for about 1 minute. Add the calamari and cook until opaque, stirring occasionally, about 4–5 minutes. Add the tomato paste and mix well for 1 minute. Add the wine and cook, stirring often, until the liquid has evaporated, about 20 minutes.

---

*U.S.-farmed freshwater prawns are raised in small-scale operations using practices that are compatible with the prawns' biology. These factors make U.S.-farmed freshwater prawns a seafood Best Choice. There are many varieties of wild-caught prawns. Do not purchase prawns from the Gulf of Mexico. If you can, convince your grocery store to purchase Australian prawns.
[†]Farmed mussels are a Best Choice because they are farmed in an environmentally responsible way.

Add the tomatoes and juice to the calamari and season with salt and pepper to taste. The squid should be tender. Stir in the fish stock, butter, snapper, and the shrimp, then place the mussels evenly over the top. Cook covered, without stirring, until the snapper is just cooked and the mussels have opened, about 10 minutes. Discard any unopened mussels.

To serve the stew, ladle into large, white bowls with wide rims placing the seafood in each bowl and covering with the broth. To garnish, drizzle the top of the stew with a little olive oil.

Pan-seared Salmon with
Avocado Slices & Lime Dressing

SERVES 2

This salmon recipe is very simple and takes just minutes to make.
The avocado complements the salmon perfectly. For a light dinner,
serve this dish with a salad of grapefruit and microgreens.

The Fish

> 2 3-ounce pieces wild-caught Alaskan salmon
> escalopes
> ½ teaspoon sea salt and a twist of pepper
> 2 tablespoons coconut oil or cold-pressed sesame oil
> 1 avocado, pit removed and sliced
> Garnish: ½ cup organic cherry tomatoes, halved,
> generous sprigs of watercress

The Lime Dressing

> 2 tablespoons extra-virgin olive oil
> 3 tablespoons white onion, finely minced
> 2 tablespoons cilantro leaves, chopped
> 2 to 3 teaspoons jalapeños, seeded and finely diced
> 1 tablespoon fresh lime juice
> pinch of sea salt

Season the escalopes with the salt and pepper. Place on a plate while preparing the dressing.

For the lime dressing: Whisk together the dressing ingredients in a bowl. Set aside.

For the fish: In a heavy-bottomed skillet on medium-high heat, heat the oil. Sear the salmon for 1–2 minutes on each side.

To serve: Place the salmon on the dinner plates and top with the avocado slices and the lime dressing. Garnish with the cherry tomatoes and watercress.

GRASSFED
MEATS

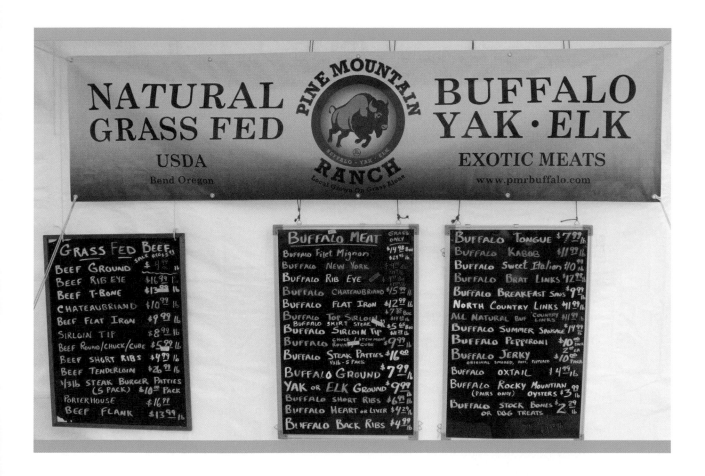

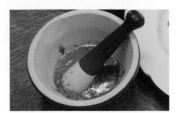

Grilled Flank Steak
with Salsa Verde

SERVES 4

This is a family dinner that will please everyone.
The steak is great with grilled or roasted vegetables and wedges
of iceberg lettuce with blue cheese dressing. Please leave time
to marinate the steak prior to grilling.

The Steak

1 pound grassfed beef flank steak

The Marinade

¾ cup extra-virgin olive oil

4 cloves garlic, minced

4 tablespoons fresh rosemary, minced

4 tablespoons fresh thyme, minced

4 tablespoons Italian (flat leaf) parsley, chopped

The Salsa Verde

1 tablespoon fresh whole oregano leaves

1 cup Italian (flat leaf) parsley, leaves only

¼ cup fresh mint leaves

¾ cup extra-virgin olive oil

1 clove garlic

1 to 2 teaspoons anchovies, chopped

1 tablespoon capers, drained

juice of ½ lemon

freshly ground pepper

For the steak: Mix the marinade ingredients in a small bowl and then pour the mixture into a 9 × 13-inch glass baking dish. Place the steak in the dish and coat both sides with the marinade. Cover with plastic wrap and refrigerate for at least 4 hours, turning the steak several times.

For the salsa verde: Place the herbs in a mortar and pestle and pound to a paste. Add a little olive oil and work it in. Transfer the mixture to a bowl. Add the garlic clove and anchovies to the mortar and pestle with a little more olive oil and pound to a paste. Add this mixture to the herbs. Crush the capers in the mortar and pestle and also add them to the rest of the ingredients. Stir in the remaining olive oil to the combined ingredients, and then stir in the lemon juice and pepper. Adjust the seasonings to achieve a balance of flavors.

To cook: Heat the grill to medium hot. With a paper towel wipe the excess marinade off the steak and place on the grill. Cook the meat for 3–4 minutes on one side, turn and cook for another 3 minutes or until done. Grassfed meat is best rare to medium rare.

Remove the steak from the grill to a cutting board and let it rest for 3–5 minutes. Slice the meat across the grain.

To serve: Place the steak slices on a platter and spoon the salsa verde over the top. Surround the steak with your grilled vegetables. Serve the lettuce wedges with the blue cheese dressing on the side.

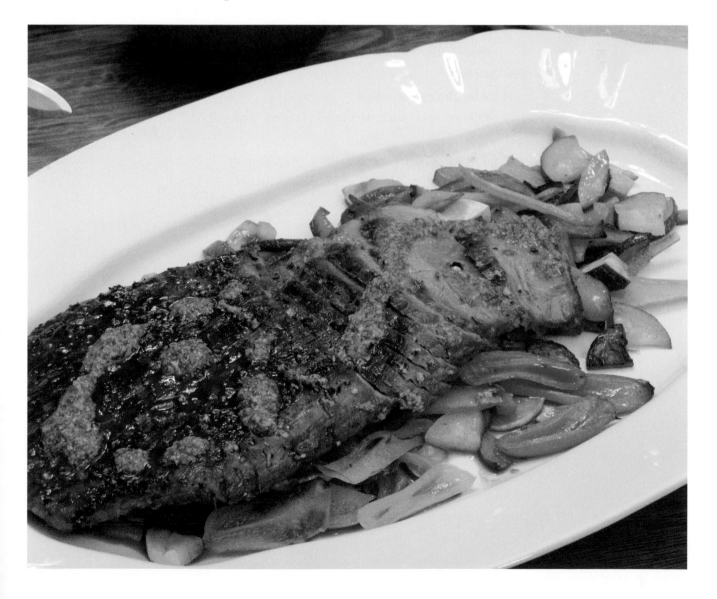

Lamb Shanks Adobo

SERVES 4

This rich recipe makes a great alternative to the traditional turkey at Thanksgiving or for a wonderful Christmas Eve dinner. Festive accompaniments would be the Sautéed Greens (page 168) and Spaghetti Squash Gratin (page 173). In addition, a fall salad of pears, pecans, and pomegranate seeds are the perfect complement.

The Lamb

4 small lamb shanks

1 teaspoon sea salt and freshly ground pepper

2 tablespoons cold-pressed sesame oil

Garnish: 2 tablespoons each, finely minced scallions and cilantro leaves

The Adobo

8 garlic cloves, unpeeled

6 dried ancho chilies, stemmed, seeded, and wiped clean

1 quart freshly squeezed organic orange juice

2 tablespoons unfiltered apple cider vinegar

2 tablespoons fresh oregano leaves

2 teaspoons sea salt

1 tablespoon ground cumin

2 tablespoons freshly ground black pepper

$\frac{1}{8}$ teaspoon ground cloves

1 cinnamon stick

2 dried bay leaves

Preheat the oven to 325 degrees.

For the lamb: Sprinkle the lamb shanks with salt and pepper. In a heavy-bottomed skillet, heat the sesame oil over medium-high heat. Brown the shanks, turning as needed, until evenly browned. Transfer the shanks to a 9 × 13-inch glass baking dish. Cover with plastic wrap while you prepare the adobo.

For the adobo: Over medium-heat in a heavy-bottomed skillet (no oil), roast the garlic cloves until light brown, stirring often, 12–15 minutes. Remove the garlic from the skillet and peel when cool. Add the chilies to the skillet, toasting until fragrant and turning them on all sides, being careful not to burn them. Add the orange juice and all the other adobo ingredients, including the peeled garlic, to the skillet. Bring the ingredients to a soft boil, then cover and simmer for about 10 minutes. Remove and save the cinnamon stick and bay leaves and set the adobo aside to cool. When cool, puree the adobo in a blender until smooth.

To finish preparing the shanks: Pour off the oil from the skillet and then add the pureed adobo along with the cinnamon and bay leaves. Bring the mixture to a boil while stirring. Then pour the adobo over the lamb shanks and add additional water to cover the shanks. Cover the baking dish with aluminum foil and seal tightly. Bake the shanks for 2 hours, turning once. Shanks will be fork tender when done.

To serve: Remove the shanks to a warmed serving platter in the oven. Skim the fat off the adobo sauce and place it in a saucepan to reheat. Place the shanks on the dinner plates and ladle some adobo sauce over the top. Sprinkle each with the garnish of scallion and cilantro.

Tequila Beef Stew with Lime Cream & Jalapeño Cabbage Slaw

SERVES 8

This fragrantly spicy south of the border beef stew is a great party dish.
The cabbage slaw with the jalapeños is a zippy accompaniment.

The Stew

2½ to 3 pounds grassfed stew beef, cut into 2-inch cubes

2 teaspoons sea salt and freshly ground pepper

4 tablespoons cold-pressed sesame oil, divided

1 medium yellow onion, chopped

1 teaspoon chopped garlic

14 ounces organic Muir Glen or San Marzano plum
   tomatoes, chopped, juice reserved

1 tablespoon fresh oregano leaves, chopped

1 tablespoon ground cumin, toasted in a small pan

Garnish: lime cream, avocado slices (3 per person),
   cilantro sprigs, lime wedges, and crumbled sheep's
   milk feta cheese

The Braising Marinade

2 large, dried chipotle chilies

2 large, dried ancho chilies

1½ cups vegetable stock (recipe in soup section)

¼ cup tequila (silver)

The Cabbage Slaw

4 tablespoons extra-virgin olive oil

6 tablespoons finely minced white onion

4 tablespoons cilantro leaves, chopped

4 teaspoons jalapeños, seeded and finely diced

3 tablespoons fresh lime juice

pinch of sea salt

6 cups red and white cabbage, very thinly sliced

The Lime Cream

1 cup Capretta Rich and Creamy Goat Yogurt or
   Green Valley lactose-free sour cream

1 tablespoon, or more, lime juice

Preheat the oven to 350 degrees.

For the stew: Season the beef cubes with the salt and pepper. Heat 3 tablespoons of the sesame oil in a heavy-bottomed skillet over medium heat. Brown the beef very well in small batches. Transfer the meat to a bowl. In the same skillet, add the remaining sesame oil and brown the onion and garlic, about 5 minutes. Stir in the tomatoes, juice, oregano, and toasted cumin. Stir well to incorporate flavors. Set aside.

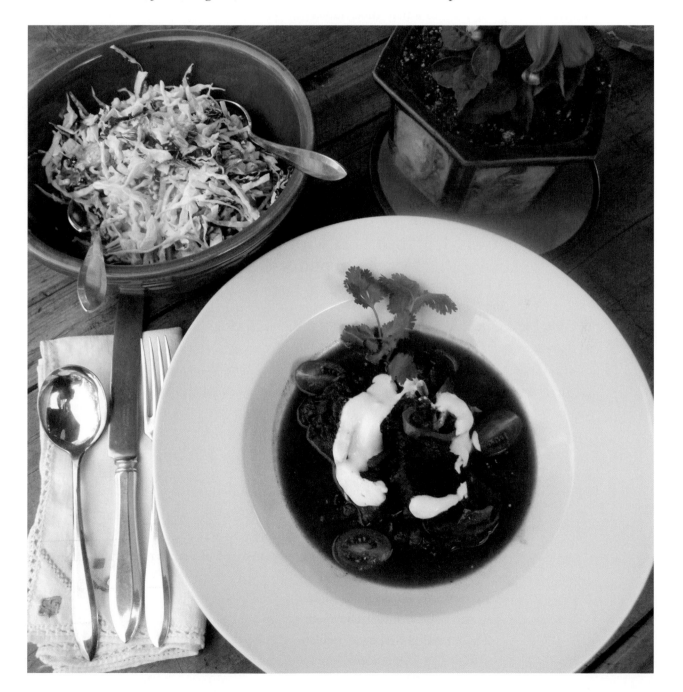

For the braising marinade: In a heavy-bottomed skillet over medium heat toast the chilies until fragrant and puffy, turning them occasionally. Set aside to cool, then remove the stems and seeds. Place the chilies in a bowl and cover with the stock and tequila. Reserve this braising mixture to add to the stew.

To finish preparing the stew: Transfer the beef mixture and the braising marinade to a large Dutch oven and add enough water to barely cover the beef. On the stove burner, heat the mixture to a boil, then transfer it to the preheated oven and cover with the lid. Bake the stew until very tender, about 3 hours.

For the slaw: Whisk all the ingredients, except for the cabbage, in a bowl. Just prior to serving, toss the dressing with the sliced cabbage in a large bowl.

For the lime cream: Mix the yogurt and lime juice in a bowl. Set aside to use as a garnish.

To serve: Skim the fat off the top of the braising liquid. Ladle the stew into large soup bowls and swirl the lime cream on top. Garnish with the avocado slices, cilantro, crumbled feta, and lime wedges. Serve the slaw on the side.

Grassfed Meat Loaf with Cauliflower "Mashed Potatoes"

SERVES 6

Meat loaf and mashed potatoes were always on the menu when I was growing up. I am sure your family will find this version fun, with the eggs in the middle of the loaf. The Cauliflower "Mashed Potatoes" (page 166) are better than the real thing. To complete the meal serve the meat loaf with an abundant salad.

The Meat Loaf

½ cup pastured cream, goat's milk, or almond milk

1 pastured egg, slightly beaten

1 teaspoon sea salt and several grinds of pepper

½ teaspoon dry mustard

1 tablespoon aged balsamic vinegar

1 cup very finely chopped almonds (instead of breadcrumbs)

1½ pounds grassfed ground beef

1 cup thinly sliced mushrooms

½ cup yellow onion, chopped

2 to 3 hard-boiled eggs, peeled

The Glaze

    4 tablespoons Grilled Tomato Ketchup (page 153) or
       organic ketchup
    1 tablespoon aged balsamic vinegar

Preheat the oven to 350 degrees.

For the meat loaf: In a large bowl combine the cream, beaten egg, salt and pepper, dry mustard, balsamic vinegar, and finely chopped almonds. Let the mixture stand for about 5 minutes and then add the ground beef, mushrooms, and onion. Mix to incorporate all ingredients. In a 9 × 13-inch glass baking dish, shape the meat mixture into a loaf, placing the hard-boiled eggs in the center.

For the glaze: After one hour of baking mix, the glaze ingredients—the ketchup and balsamic vinegar—together and brush on the meat loaf. Return to the oven for about 10 minutes.

To serve: Cool the meat loaf for about 5 minutes and then slice the portions to reveal the cross section of eggs. Place the meat loaf on the dinner plates. Pass the cauliflower "mashed potatoes" and salad.

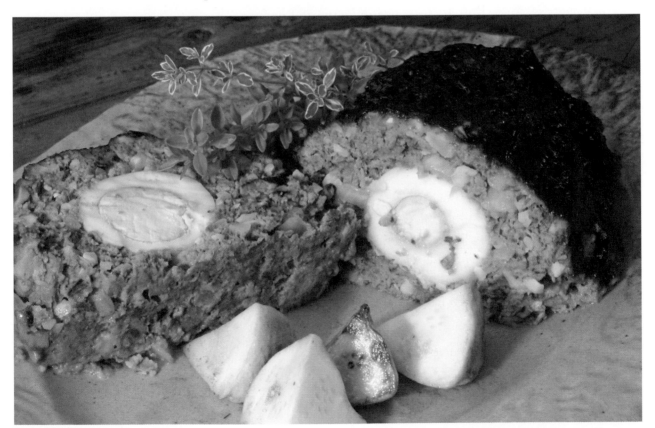

Greek Lamb Kebabs with Tzatziki

SERVES 8

Tzatziki is a traditional Greek yogurt-cucumber sauce. As an accompaniment, serve these succulent lamb kebabs with your favorite grilled vegetables and the Mediterranean Spinach and Feta Salad (page 147). For dessert, grill some figs and sprinkle them with a few drops of flavored balsamic vinegar.* Slices of late-summer melon are also perfect.

The Tzatziki

You can make the tsatziki a day in advance.

¾ cup Mediterranean cucumbers, finely diced

1 cup Capretta Rich and Creamy Goat Yogurt

1 scant teaspoon minced garlic

2 teaspoons fresh lemon juice

2 tablespoons fresh mint leaves, chopped

4 tablespoons extra-virgin olive oil

pinch of sea salt and a twist of pepper

The Kebab Marinade

2 cups hearty red wine, zinfandel is perfect

2 teaspoons dried oregano

1 tablespoon ground cumin

2 teaspoons dried thyme

1 teaspoon cinnamon

6 cloves garlic, smashed

2 teaspoons sea salt and freshly ground pepper, to
     taste

The Lamb Kebabs

2 pounds grassfed leg of lamb cut into 2-inch cubes

1 small red onion cut into 1-inch chunks

2 red bell peppers cut into 1-inch chunks

---

*For a really wonderful treat order some flavored balsamic vinegars from Olive Oil and Beyond in Newport Beach, California: www.oliveoilandbeyond.com. At our house we have chocolate, blueberry, and peach.

Garnish: 1 cup Italian (flat leaf) parsley leaves,
    chopped; 4 scallions, white and green parts, sliced
    thinly on the diagonal

For the tsatziki: Mix all the ingredients in a bowl. Taste and adjust flavors. Cover and refrigerate until ready to use.

For the marinade: In a bowl whisk together all ingredients and then add the cubed lamb. Mix well. Cover the bowl with plastic wrap and let the meat marinate at room temperature for 2 hours or in the refrigerator overnight.

For the kebabs: Turn on the grill to medium hot. You can also use your oven broiler with the rack about 7–8 inches from the flame.

Remove the lamb from the marinade. Pour the marinade into a saucepan and bring to a boil. Thread the lamb cubes on long metal skewers (4 ounces on each), alternating with the onion and red bell pepper. Season the kebabs with a sprinkle of salt and freshly ground pepper. Grill the kebabs while basting with the marinade, until they are evenly browned on all sides but still pink in the middle, about 15 minutes.

To serve: Place the kebabs on a warm platter. On the side serve the grilled vegetables and the Mediterranean Spinach and Feta Salad. Pour the tzatziki into a bowl and let your guests help themselves.

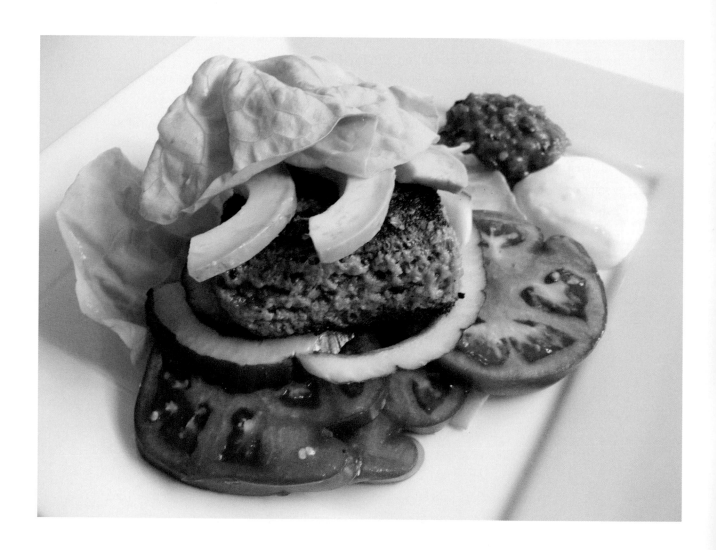

Blue Cheese Burger
on a Butter Lettuce Bun

SERVES 2

This delicious burger has no bun. You will never miss it.
What makes these burgers so tasty and moist is the caramelized onion.

4 tablespoons sesame oil, divided

2 medium yellow onions, thinly sliced

6 ounces grassfed ground beef, 3 ounces per person

2 tablespoons pastured cream or milk

1 tablespoon aged balsamic vinegar

1 tablespoon organic ketchup or gluten and soy-free
   Worcestershire sauce

¼ teaspoon sea salt and a twist of pepper

4 large leaves of red leaf butter lettuce

4 ounces Point Reyes Blue raw cow's milk cheese*

Burger garnishes: 1 garden tomato, thickly sliced,
   avocado slices, more caramelized onions

In a heavy-bottomed skillet heat 2 tablespoons of the sesame oil and slowly caramelize the onion slices until brown and creamy.

In a bowl combine the ground beef, caramelized onions (reserving ¾ of the onions for garnishing the finished burgers), cream, balsamic vinegar, and ketchup. Season with salt and a couple twists of pepper and mix well. Divide the mixture into two balls and then form into patties about ¾-inch thick.

In a heavy-bottomed skillet heat the remaining 2 tablespoons of sesame oil over medium-high heat and brown the burgers for 1–2 minutes on each side. Rare is good.

To serve: Place one large butter lettuce leaf in the center of each dinner plate. Place the burger on the lettuce leaf and top with the blue cheese, more caramelized onion, and your chosen garnishes. Place the remaining butter lettuce leaf on top of the burger.

---

*As an alternative consider Berger Basque raw sheep's milk cheese, Roquefort papillon, or Bleu du Bocage rare blue goat cheese. Humboldt Fog cheese or raw goat cheddar are also great.

Short Ribs
Braised in Zinfandel

SERVES 8

For a rich and satisfying dinner, serve these succulent short ribs with Sautéed Greens (page 168) and the Roasted Winter Vegetables (page 172). After the ribs marinate overnight, they are very simple to prepare. This is a five-star dinner.

The Ribs

8 large grassfed beef short ribs

The Short Rib Marinade

Marinate the ribs overnight.

8 tablespoons cold-pressed sesame oil, divided

1 cup chopped onions

½ cup leeks, chopped and rinsed of any grit

1 Granny Smith apple, chopped

6 cloves garlic

2 jalapeños, seeded and diced

4 cups Zinfandel (omit the wine and use vegetable broth if you cannot have wine)

4 fresh thyme sprigs

4 fresh sage leaves

1 teaspoon coriander seeds, wrapped in cheesecloth

sea salt and freshly ground pepper, to taste

4 cups vegetable stock (recipe in soup section)

For the marinade: In a large sauté pan heat 4 tablespoons of the sesame oil and caramelize the onions, leeks, apple, garlic, and jalapeños for 7–10 minutes. Add the Zinfandel and bring the mixture to a simmer. Remove from the heat and cool. Transfer the mixture to a large, rectangular glass baking dish and place the short ribs in the marinade. Add the thyme sprigs, sage leaves, and coriander seeds wrapped in the cheesecloth. Season the ribs with salt and pepper. Coat the ribs very well with the marinade mixture, cover with plastic wrap, and refrigerate for 24 hours.

To cook: Heat the oven to 350 degrees. Remove the short ribs from the marinade and pat very dry with paper towels. In a heavy-bottomed skillet, sear the short ribs in the remaining 4 tablespoons of oil for 2–3 minutes on each side, or until nicely browned. Place the ribs in a roasting pan and cover with the marinade and the vegetable stock. Cover with foil and braise 3–4 hours until the meat is fork tender.

Remove the roasting pan from the oven and turn off the oven. Place the ribs in a baking dish, cover, and keep in the warm oven. Strain the braising juices into a saucepan and reduce the sauce to 1½ cups.

To serve: Place the sautéed greens in the center of the dinner plates. Place one rib on top of the greens. Surround the ribs with some of the roasted vegetables. Spoon the reduced sauce generously over the ribs.

Braised Short Ribs
with Cauliflower Puree, Brussels Sprouts
& Caramelized Apples

SERVES 6

I have to tell you this meal is completely worth the effort
and will make a marvelous holiday dinner in place of the more traditional fare.
To make the holiday preparations easier, you can prepare the short ribs
and the cauliflower puree a day in advance.

The Short Ribs

6 large grassfed boneless beef short ribs

pinch of sea salt and freshly ground pepper

2 tablespoons cold-pressed sesame oil

The Short Rib Braising Liquid

2 tablespoons cold-pressed sesame oil

1 carrot, small dice

1 medium onion, chopped

3 organic Muir Glen or San Marzano plum tomatoes, chopped

2 cups pinot noir (use Hearty Vegetable Stock on
  page 103 if you cannot have wine)

4 bay leaves

1 teaspoon peppercorns

2 quarts Hearty Vegetable Stock

Cauliflower Puree (prepare a day in advance)

Use the Cauliflower "Mashed Potato" recipe (page
  166), thinned

Pastured cream for thinning

Brussels Sprouts, Bacon & Caramelized Apples

15 Brussels sprouts, cut into fourths

8 ounces Beeler's Humanely Raised Organic Bacon,
  diced

3 Granny Smith apples, peeled and cut into eighths

The Apple Salad Garnish

1 Granny Smith apple, julienned

1 ounce fresh horseradish, grated

3 small celery leaves
olive oil
lemon juice
pinch of sea salt and ground pepper

Preheat the oven to 300 degrees.

For the short ribs: First salt and pepper the ribs. In a large skillet, heat the sesame oil and sear the meat on all sides until evenly browned. Set aside.

For the braising liquid: Wipe out the skillet with a paper towel and add more sesame oil. With the heat on medium, add the chopped vegetables and sauté until lightly browned. Add the pinot noir and reduce to ¼ of the original liquid amount. Add the bay leaves, peppercorns, and the vegetable stock. Simmer the mixture for about 25 minutes.

To cook the ribs: Place the ribs in a large Dutch oven or roasting pan. Pour the braising liquid over the short ribs, leaving plenty of room for the ribs. Bake ribs for 3 hours or until fork tender. If you cook the ribs a day in advance and refrigerate overnight, you can easily skim off the fat prior to reheating the ribs. Reheat the ribs in the oven, covered in foil, in some of the braising liquid.

For the Brussels sprouts: Place the bacon in a small saucepan and cover with water. Simmer for 45 minutes. Drain. Blanch Brussels sprouts in lightly salted water until bright green and slightly tender. Add blanched bacon pieces to a large skillet and sauté until crisp. Add the apple slices and cook slowly until browned and caramelized, adding a little sesame oil if necessary. Toss in the Brussels sprouts just before serving and mix ingredients well.

To finish the dinner: Remove the ribs from the braising liquid, skimming off as much fat as possible. Strain the braising liquid into a saucepan and reduce over high heat until the mixture coats a spoon and is very thick. Pour the sauce over the reheated ribs to glaze.

Reheat and thin the cauliflower puree with the addition of cream. Bring the sauce of the reheated ribs to a boil. Have your Brussels sprouts and apple salad garnish ready in a bowl.

For the apple salad garnish: Toss the listed ingredients in a bowl. Use just a drizzle of olive oil and a couple drops of lemon juice.

Plate assembly: On each plate paint a swath of the cauliflower puree. Place a short rib over the puree. Scatter the Brussels sprouts and caramelized apples around the plate. Spoon the heated sauce over the ribs. Top the short ribs with the apple salad.

South of the Border Pork Stew

SERVES 8–10

What could be more festive? This wonderful pork stew has all the spicy flavors of Mexico that I love. Pork shoulder is inexpensive, but the preparation here makes it special enough for company. I served it for our Christmas dinner with roasted vegetables, Spaghetti Squash Gratin (page 173), and Mexican Cole Slaw with Chipotle-Lime Dressing (page 150). You can cook the stew in the slow cooker, which is my favorite way of making this dish.

The Dry Marinade
Marinate the pork overnight.

1 tablespoon ground cumin seeds, toasted

2 tablespoons ground coriander

2 tablespoons crushed fennel seed

1 teaspoon cayenne

6 cloves garlic, chopped

1 tablespoon fresh oregano leaves

1 tablespoon fresh thyme leaves

The Pork

3 pounds pork* shoulder, cut into 2-inch chunks

The Pork Stew

4 tablespoons cold-pressed sesame oil

1 cup sweet onion, chopped

¼ cup carrot, peeled and diced

¼ cup diced fennel

2 bay leaves

1 teaspoon red chili flakes

1 cup dry white wine (optional)

4 cups chicken stock or vegetable stock (recipes in
   soup section)

zest of 1 lemon (long strips of zest)

4 sprigs cilantro

---

*Try the Llano Seco or Beeler's brand humanely raised organic pork.

sea salt and freshly ground pepper
Garnish: pomegranate seeds (available in the fall),
   1 cup cilantro leaves

For the marinade: Combine the marinade ingredients in a large bowl and then mix in the pork chunks. Cover and refrigerate overnight. Let the meat warm to room temperature before cooking, about 45 minutes. Season the meat with salt and pepper. Save the garlic and herbs to add to the stew later.

For the pork: Preheat the oven to 325 degrees. In a large sauté pan, heat the sesame oil over medium heat. Add the pork in batches and brown evenly on all sides. Remove the browned pork to a plate.

After browning the meat, pour off excess oil from the sauté pan and add the onion, carrot, and fennel. Stir well to incorporate all the browned bits left in the pan. Cook until the vegetables are nicely caramelized. Add the white wine and reduce by half, about 5 minutes. Add the chicken stock.

Add the pork back into the mixture along with the garlic, herbs, spices, and lemon zest. Transfer the stew to your slow cooker, turned to high. Make sure the liquid covers the meat. Add a little water if necessary. Cook the stew until fork tender, about 3 hours. If you are cooking the stew in the oven, transfer it to a Dutch oven with a lid. Braise in the oven for about 2½ hours.

To finish the preparation: Remove the pork from the braising liquid and strain it into a saucepan. Put the pork in a large glass baking dish. Turn the oven up to 400 degrees and place the pork in the oven to caramelize a little, about 15 minutes, while you reduce the sauce. Reduce the sauce until it is thickened and slightly coats the back of a spoon.

To serve: Place the pork stew in a deep serving dish surrounded by the roasted vegetables. Sprinkle the pomegranate seeds and chopped cilantro on top. Serve the spaghetti squash gratin and the coleslaw on the side. Pass the sauce in a gravy boat.

Lamb Chops with Cumin Yogurt & Oregano Pesto

SERVES 4

I love the fragrant and exotic flavors of the Middle East. These lamb chops are succulent and delicious. Serve them with a spinach, cucumber, red onion, and feta salad and some grilled tomatoes and eggplant. Wow!

The Lamb Chops

2 to 3 lamb rib chops* per person, cut into chops

Lamb Chop Marinade

Marinate lamb for 4 hours.

¼ cup fresh mint leaves, finely chopped

2 tablespoons extra-virgin olive oil

zest of 1 lemon

1 teaspoon sea salt and a twist of pepper

The Cumin Yogurt

1 tablespoon cumin seeds, toasted (toast briefly in a small sauté pan)

1 cup Capretta Rich and Creamy Goat Yogurt

1 tablespoon extra-virgin olive oil

1 tablespoon lemon juice

pinch of sea salt and a twist of pepper

The Oregano Pesto

2 cups fresh oregano leaves, preferably from the garden

pinch of sea salt and a twist of pepper

¼ cup, or more, extra-virgin olive oil

Garnish: zest of 2 lemons (cut very finely in long strips, using a lemon zester) and sprigs of fresh mint

For the marinade: In the bowl of a food processor blend the marinade ingredients (mint, olive oil, lemon zest, salt, and pepper) until a rough paste is formed. Rub the marinade over both sides of the lamb chops and place them in a rectangular glass

---

*Try the New Zealand grassfed rack of lamb at Trader Joe's.

baking dish. It's best to marinate the chops for about 4 hours to let the flavors infuse into the meat. Refrigerate until ready to cook.

For the cumin yogurt: Crush the toasted cumin seeds in a mortar and pestle. Mix the remaining ingredients in a small bowl. Cover and refrigerate until ready to use.

For the oregano pesto: Place the ingredients, except for the olive oil, in a food processor. With the motor running, slowly add the olive oil until well blended into a smooth paste. Remove the pesto to a bowl and cover with a thin cap of olive oil. Cover the bowl with plastic wrap until ready to use.

To cook: Preheat the grill or broiler. Cook the chops rare to medium rare, 4–5 minutes on each side. When the lamb chops are done remove them to a platter and let them rest while you prepare to plate the dinner.

To serve: Overlap the lamb chops on each dinner plate and arrange the grilled tomatoes and eggplant on the side. Drizzle the cumin yogurt sauce around the mound of chops, and then drizzle the oregano pesto around the plate. Garnish the lamb chops with the lemon zest and sprigs of fresh mint. Serve the salad on separate plates.

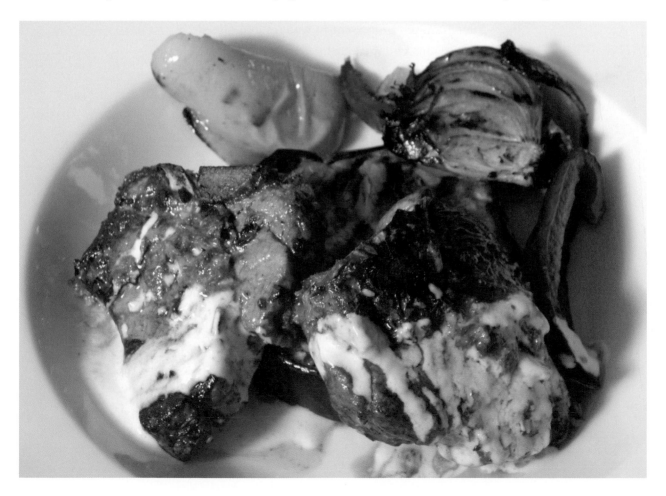

Flat Iron Fajitas on
Butter Lettuce "Tortillas"
with Colorful Sweet Peppers

SERVES 4

Flat iron is a very flavorful and less-expensive cut of steak and is now showing up on menus around the country. This dish tastes best when you can use colorful peppers from your garden or interesting peppers from the farmers' market. To eliminate grains from the recipe, I've substituted large leaves of red butter lettuce for the usual tortillas. This alternative is both fun and delicious.

The Flat Iron Steak

1 pound grassfed flat iron steak, thinly sliced (3
   ounces per person)
sea salt and freshly ground pepper

The Fajita Filling

4 cups colorful peppers, seeded and thinly sliced
1 medium red onion, cut in wedges and sliced
4 teaspoons chopped garlic
6 tablespoons sesame oil, divided
juice of 1 lime
sea salt

The Lime Cream

1 cup Capretta's Rich and Creamy Goat Yogurt or
   lactose-free sour cream
1 tablespoon fresh lime juice
Garnish: chopped cilantro, additional wedges of
   lime, guacamole or sliced avocados, grated sheep's
   milk manchego, your favorite salsa, diced garden
   tomatoes or organic cherry tomatoes, halved

The Fajita "Tortillas"

1 head red leaf butter lettuce, washed and dried

Prepare the steak: Season the steak with salt and pepper. Place the steak in a baking dish, cover, and let sit while preparing the other ingredients.

   Prepare the chopped vegetables and garlic: in a large skillet sauté the peppers, onion, and garlic in 3 tablespoons of the sesame oil until they reach the desired doneness, adding salt "to taste" while cooking. Add the lime juice and set the vegetables aside in a baking dish in a warm oven.

Prepare the lime cream: In a bowl mix together the yogurt and the lime juice.

Prepare the garnishes: Place garnish ingredients in separate bowls.

For the fajitas: When you are ready to prepare the fajitas, place your butter lettuce tortillas on 4 dinner plates (two for each person).

In another skillet with the remaining 3 tablespoons of oil, quickly sauté the steak slices over high heat, cooking until just barely done and still showing some pink. Remove the steak from the pan immediately to stop the cooking. You may also grill the steak slices.

To serve: Arrange the vegetables evenly over the lettuce tortillas. Divide the steak equally as well. Drizzle the steak with some lime cream and chopped cilantro. Place the lime wedges on each plate. Let everyone help themselves to the remaining garnishes.

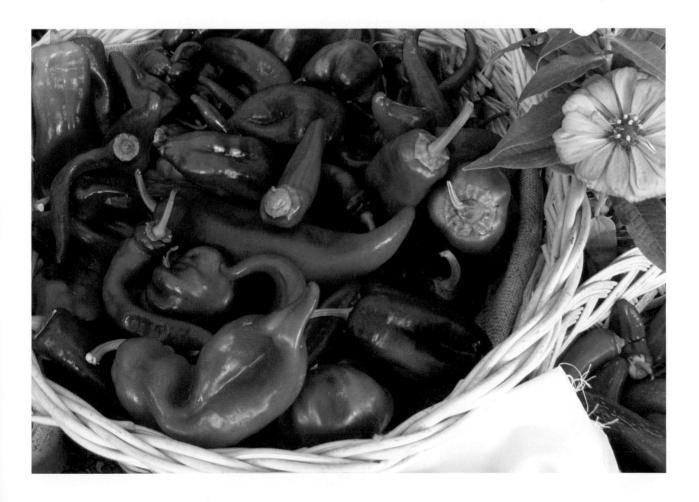

Grilled Rib-Eye Steak with Dry Steak Rub

SERVES 4

You will want to marinate the rib eye for 24 hours prior to cooking. The steak is perfect with grilled vegetables. Serve with a Caesar salad or a wedge of crisp iceberg lettuce and Blue Cheese Dressing (page 120). You could not get a better dinner in a fine restaurant.

The Dry Steak Rub
Marinate the steak overnight.

- 3 tablespoons ground cumin
- 2 tablespoons freshly ground pepper
- 2 tablespoons Chimayo chili powder
- 1 tablespoon garlic powder
- 1 tablespoon fennel seed
- 1 tablespoon ground coriander
- 1 tablespoon sea salt

The Steak

- 1 pound grassfed boneless rib-eye steak (about 4 ounces per person), 1½ inches thick

The Olive Oil and Balsamic Vinegar Sauce

- 1 tablespoon minced shallot or white part of scallion
- ¼ cup extra-virgin olive oil
- 2 to 3 tablespoons aged balsamic vinegar

To marinate the beef: In a small bowl combine the ingredients and mix well. Rub a portion of the mixture liberally over the steak on both sides. Reserve any of the remaining rub for another use. After coating the steak with the rub, wrap it in plastic and refrigerate for 24 hours.

For the balsamic vinegar sauce: Whisk the shallot, oil, and vinegar together. Set aside.

To grill the steak: Preheat the grill to medium hot. Remove the rib eye from the refrigerator and wipe off excess steak rub with a paper towel. Grill or broil the meat to rare or medium rare, turning the steak over every 5 minutes or so. Remove the meat to a cutting board and let rest for about 5 minutes before slicing.

To serve: Place your grilled vegetables on a platter, leaving room in the middle for the steak slices. Slice the steak thinly across the grain and place the slices on the platter. Spoon the olive oil and balsamic sauce over everything. Serve the salad on the side. Let the guests help themselves.

PASTURED POULTRY

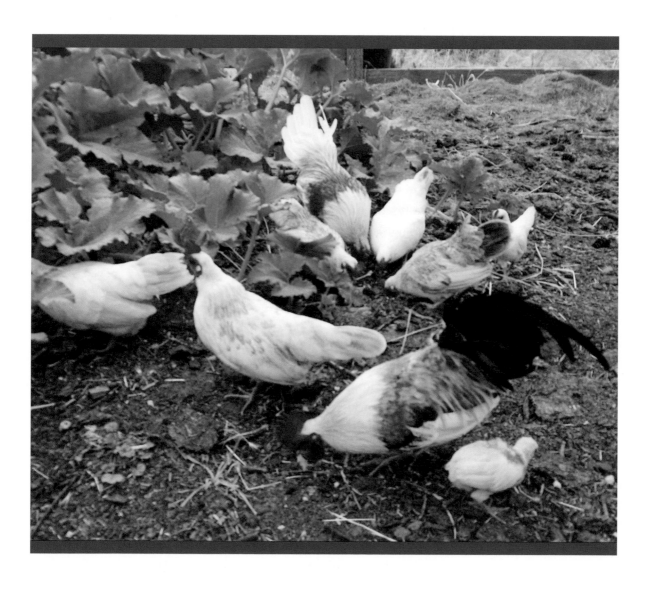

Asian Chicken Meatballs with
Stir-Fried Vegetables

SERVES 6

These meatballs are delicious and easy to make. Served with the stir-fried vegetables and the flavorful dipping sauce, they make a fun family dinner. You can also prepare the Asian Cauliflower "Fried Rice" (see page 162) for an additional accompaniment.

The Chicken Meatballs

2 ounces fresh ginger, peeled and roughly chopped

1½ pounds organic boneless pastured or organic chicken thighs, cut into small pieces

Stevita, stevia (a very small amount, to taste), optional

2 teaspoons coconut flour

1 teaspoon sea salt

½ teaspoon white pepper

sesame oil or coconut oil for frying (make sure you have enough)

Garnish: 1 cup cilantro leaves, chopped; toasted sesame seeds

The Stir-Fried Vegetables

The following are suggestions—choose your favorites!

4 tablespoons cold-pressed sesame oil

1 cup shiitake mushrooms, thinly sliced

4 cloves garlic, chopped

1 cup Brussels sprouts, halved

3 to 4 scallions, white and green parts, sliced on the diagonal

3 heads baby bok choi, cut lengthwise into quarters

2 red bell peppers, seeded and thinly sliced

2 cups snow peas (add at the very end of cooking)

pinch of sea salt

The Asian Dipping Sauce

Prepare sauce in advance.

> 2 tablespoons Rapunzel non-GMO organic corn starch
>
> ¼ cup Coconut Secret Coconut Aminos (more if desired)
>
> ¼ cup dry marsala wine
>
> Stevita, to taste (very small amount)
>
> 3 tablespoons rice wine vinegar
>
> 3 tablespoons Mirin, Japanese cooking wine

For the meatballs: Pulse the ginger in a food processor until finely diced. Add the chicken, stevia, coconut flour, salt, and white pepper. Pulse the mixture until it is a rough texture. Do not overprocess the ingredients.

In a deep sauté pan, pour the sesame oil to a depth of 3 inches. Heat the oil to 350 degrees (use a candy thermometer). Form the meatball mixture into balls about 2 inches in diameter. Drop the meatballs into the hot oil in batches and deep-fry until evenly browned, about 1–2 minutes (test for doneness). Transfer the meatballs to a paper towel–lined plate. Keep warm.

For the stir-fried vegetables: In a very large sauté pan or wok, heat the sesame oil until hot. Toss in the shiitake mushrooms and garlic and stir-fry for 1 minute then add the remaining vegetables. Season with a pinch of salt. Continue cooking the vegetables until they are done to your liking. I like them a little crisp.

For the Asian dipping sauce: In a small bowl combine the corn starch with 2 tablespoons cold water and mix well. Set aside. In a small saucepan, bring the coconut aminos, marsala, Stevita, rice wine vinegar, and Mirin to a boil and simmer for 3 minutes. Add the corn starch mixture a little at a time while whisking the sauce until it is a smooth consistency and coats the back of a spoon.

To serve: Divide the vegetable mixture onto 6 plates. Top with the meatballs and drizzle the sauce evenly over the meatballs and the vegetables. Garnish with the chopped cilantro and sesame seeds. Pass additional sauce.

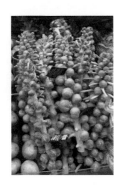

Sunday Roast Chicken with Herb Butter & Roasted Vegetables

SERVES 6

We used to have roast chicken every Sunday when I was growing up. Roast chicken is family comfort food. With this meal, you can put everything in the roasting pan and relax while dinner cooks. What could be more comforting than that? A nice accompaniment is the Savory Green Salad (page 124).

The Herb Compound Butter

  4 ounces pastured butter or goat butter

  1 teaspoon garlic, minced

  4 tablespoons total fresh rosemary, parsley, and
     oregano leaves, chopped

  1 teaspoon sea salt

  ½ teaspoon freshly ground pepper

  juice of 1 lemon

  zest of 1 lemon

The Chicken

  1 4-pound pastured (if available) or organic chicken,
     rinsed and patted dry

The Roasted Vegetables

  1 small cauliflower, cut into florets

  1 large yellow onion, peeled and cut into 6 wedges

  2 fennel bulbs, sliced

  ½ cup white wine or chicken stock (recipe for stock
     in soup section)

  1 tablespoon fennel seeds, crushed in morter

  a few sprigs of thyme

  12 cloves garlic, crushed

  1 pound Brussels sprouts, cleaned of outer leaves

  1 pound shiitake mushrooms, tough stems removed
     (or small brown mushrooms left whole)

  12 large sage leaves

  juice of one lemon

  2 tablespoons sesame oil

sea salt and freshly ground pepper
1 tablespoon coconut flour (for making the sauce)
Garnish: juice of 1 lemon; ½ cup parsley leaves, chopped

Preheat the oven to 400 degrees.

For the compound butter: In a small bowl mix the butter, garlic, herbs, salt, pepper, lemon juice, and zest.

For the chicken: Carefully slide your hand between the skin on the breast of the chicken and the flesh to make a pocket, being careful not to break the skin. Spread one-half of the herbed butter liberally over the inside pocket of the chicken. Then rub the remaining butter over the entire outside of the chicken. Season the outside of the chicken with a little salt and pepper. Tie the legs together with kitchen string and place the chicken on a roasting rack in a large roasting pan. Arrange the cauliflower, onion, and fennel bulbs around the chicken.

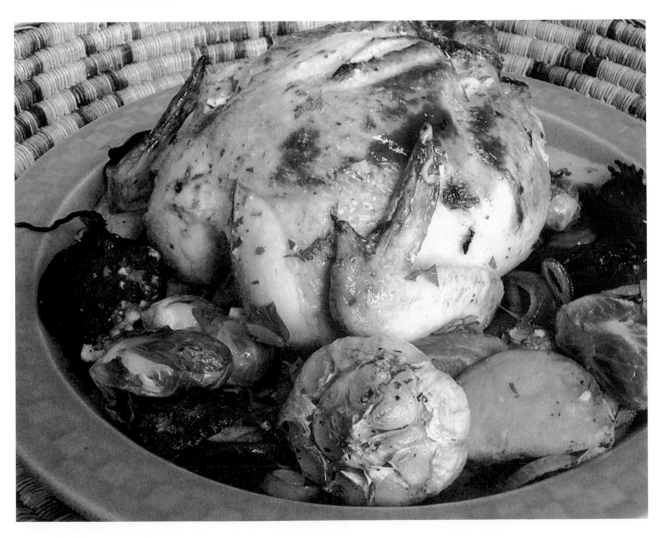

Roast the chicken for 30 minutes and then pour the wine over the top. Lower the oven temperature to 350.

For the roasted vegetables: In a large bowl mix the fennel seeds, thyme sprigs, garlic, Brussels sprouts, shiitaki mushrooms, onions, sage leaves, lemon juice, and sesame oil. Season the vegetable mixture with a little salt and pepper and add to the roasting pan. Continue roasting another 1–1½ hours, basting the chicken and vegetables every 20 minutes or so.

To finish: Test to see if the chicken is done by sticking the tip of a sharp knife between the leg and the body of the chicken where the joint attaches, making sure the juice runs clear and is not bloody. Transfer the chicken and the vegetables to a large platter on top of the stove and cover with foil to keep warm.

While the chicken is resting, pour the pan juices into a saucepan and bring to a simmer. Mix the tablespoon of coconut flour with a little water to make a paste and then whisk this into the sauce and cook for 10 minutes. If the sauce is too thick, thin with a little water or wine. Add a little salt to the sauce, if necessary.

To serve: Carve the chicken, or place it whole on the platter surrounded by the roasted vegetables. Squeeze the lemon juice over the chicken and vegetables, followed by a sprinkle of chopped parsley leaves. Pass the sauce. Serve the salad on the side.

Pineapple Red Curry Duck

SERVES 4

This is a gorgeous red curry, and with the addition of fresh pineapple it makes an absolutely mouthwatering dish. If you can, purchase one of the whole roasted ducks in an Asian market and ask them to cut it up for you. Otherwise, use cooked duck breast. A simple salad of lightly dressed greens will complement the meal.

2½ cups coconut milk, divided

¼ cup Thai Mae Ploy* red curry paste

3 cups cooked duck, cut into bite-size pieces (you
    can also use cooked chicken or pork roast)

juice and zest of 1 lime

1 cup chicken or vegetable stock (recipe in soup section)

¼ cup water

sea salt, to taste

1 cup ripe pineapple, cored, peeled, and cut into 1-inch chunks

½ cup red bell pepper, seeded and thinly sliced

2 to 3 Thai chilies or jalapeños, seeded and very finely sliced

20 organic cherry tomatoes, left whole

10 Thai basil leaves

Garnish: sprigs of cilantro

In a large saucepan over medium heat, slightly reduce 1 cup of the coconut milk, about 5 minutes. Whisk in the red curry paste and continue to simmer for another 5 minutes.

Add the cooked duck to the coconut milk–curry mixture, stirring gently until heated through, about 5 minutes.

Add the remaining coconut milk, lime juice, lime zest, stock, and water. Increase the heat and simmer until the flavors meld, about 2 minutes.

Add the salt, pineapple, red bell pepper, and chilies and continue to cook until the pineapple is tender, 3–4 minutes. Just before serving, toss in the tomatoes and basil so they retain their flavor and color.

To serve, ladle the curry into large bowls. Garnish with the cilantro sprigs. Serve the salad on a separate plate.

---

*The Mae Ploy curry paste contains shrimp paste, dried red chili, garlic, shallot, galangal, kaffir, lime peel, salt, and pepper. No MSG, preservatives, or artificial color. This is my favorite brand, available at Asian markets.

Chicken "Scallopini" with Lemon-Caper Sauce

SERVES 6

This is one of my favorite recipes for chicken breasts because it's so moist and very easy to prepare! Serve with steamed haricots verts or asparagus and a simple green salad.

The Chicken

1 cup coconut flour or almond flour (I use a mix of both)

1 cup grated sheep's milk pecorino romano or Parmesan Cheese Substitute (page 152)

6 tablespoons parsley leaves, chopped

1 tablespoon fresh rosemary, chopped

2 eggs, beaten

3 6-ounce boneless and skinless pastured or organic chicken breasts, cut in half and pounded flat

sea salt and freshly ground pepper, to taste

6 tablespoons cold-pressed sesame oil

The Lemon-Caper Sauce

To be prepared in the sauté pan.

splash of white wine (less than ¼ cup)

2 cloves of garlic, minced

juice of 1 lemon

2 tablespoons capers, rinsed

6 tablespoons pastured butter or goat butter

Turn the oven on to warm. In a glass pie pan mix the flour, cheese, parsley, and rosemary. Place the beaten eggs in another glass pie pan.

Dredge the chicken breasts, first in the beaten eggs and then in the flour mix. Season the breasts with salt and pepper then set them aside on a plate.

In a large sauté pan over medium high heat, heat the sesame oil. Sauté each breast until golden brown on each side. Add a little more oil to the pan if necessary. Remove the cooked breasts to a baking dish and place in the prewarmed oven.

To finish the lemon-caper sauce: In the same pan that you sautéed the chicken breasts, with the heat on medium high, deglaze the pan drippings with the splash of wine, less than ¼ cup. Add the garlic, lemon juice, and the capers and whisk to incorporate. Reduce the liquid volume to ½ and then whisk in the butter. When the sauce coats the back of a spoon, immediately remove from heat. You may need to add more butter if the sauce isn't thick enough. Then pour sauce into a bowl and keep warm on the stove.

To serve: Remove the breasts from the oven and place them on a cutting board. Slice the breasts on the diagonal. Fan the chicken slices on the dinner plates and spoon the lemon-caper sauce over the top. Place your vegetables on the plate on top of the chicken slices. Serve the salad on separate plates.

Baked Cilantro Chicken
with Tomato-Avocado Salsa

SERVES 6

For a very easy-to-prepare, quick dinner, this dish is the answer.
These are the fresh and vibrant Mexican flavors I love.
To complete the meal serve the chicken with Caesar Salad.

The Chicken

3 6-ounce organic chicken breasts, bone and skin
    removed, halved

The Cilantro-Lime Marinade

¼ cup extra-virgin olive oil

¼ cup lime juice

1 tablespoon ground cumin

½ cup cilantro, chopped

pinch of sea salt and a twist of pepper

Tomato-Avocado Salsa

Prepare salsa at least one hour prior to serving to give it time to chill.

2 baskets organic cherry tomatoes, halved

2 jalapeños, seeded and thinly sliced

½ cup scallions, white and green part, thinly sliced

4 tablespoons microplaned ginger

2 tablespoons garlic

2 teaspoons yellow mustard seeds

1 teaspoon red chili flakes

½ cup cold-pressed sesame oil

½ cup coconut vinegar or Champagne vinegar

3 large avocados diced into chunks

1 teaspoon sea salt and a twist of fresh pepper

Garnish: sprigs of cilantro

In a large bowl whisk together the olive oil, lime juice, cumin, cilantro, salt, and pepper. Place the chicken breasts in a 9 × 13-inch glass baking dish. Pour the marinade over the breasts, turning once to coat. Let stand for 1 hour, turning the breasts occasionally.

To prepare the tomato-avocado salsa: In a bowl combine the tomatoes, jalapeños, and scallions. In another bowl combine the ginger, garlic, and the dry spices. In a small saucepan, heat the sesame oil over medium heat, add the dry spices and cook for 1 minute. Then add the vinegar, salt, and pepper. Pour the hot mixture over the tomato mixture in the bowl. Cover and chill the salsa for at least 1 hour or for up to 4 hours. Just before serving add the avocadoes and mix well.

For the chicken: Preheat oven to 350 degrees. Remove the chicken breasts from the marinade and discard the marinade. Bake the breasts for 20 minutes, until no longer pink in the center.

To serve: Remove the breasts from the oven, cut in half, and place on dinner plates. Spoon the tomato-avocado salsa on top of the breasts. Garnish with sprigs of cilantro, if desired. Pass the Caesar salad.

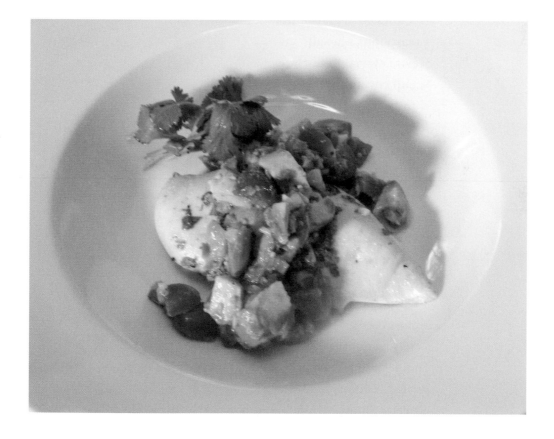

Pad Thai

SERVES 8 GENEROUSLY

This is an extravagant and colorful dinner with complex Thai flavors. If you make this recipe, you can have your Thai dinner at home each week. The Pad Thai also makes a great party buffet dish. I have removed the standard rice noodles from this recipe. If you must have noodles, try using the Zucchini Noodles (page 170), Baked Spaghetti Squash (page 173), or kelp noodles.*

Pad Thai Sauce

You can prepare the sauce the day before. Makes over 2 cups.

- 3 ounces preserved tamarind paste (Asian market or section of grocery store)
- 10 tablespoons hot water
- 4 teaspoons sea salt
- Stevita stevia, to taste
- ¾ cup coconut vinegar
- ¾ to 1 cup water

The Salad

- ½ head savoy cabbage, core removed
- 4 tablespoons cold-pressed sesame oil
- 4 tablespoons dried shrimp (from the Asian section of your grocery store)
- ½ teaspoon red chili flakes
- ¼ cup carrots, cut into matchsticks
- ¼ cup red bell pepper, thinly sliced
- 3 teaspoons minced garlic
- 3 cups cooked fish or shrimp, shells removed (or leftover shredded chicken or beef)
- 1 tablespoon Coconut Secret Raw Coconut Aminos
- juice of 2 limes
- 6 to 8 scallions, white and green parts, thinly sliced on the diagonal

---

*Kelp noodles are a sea vegetable in the form of an easy-to-prepare noodle. Prepare according to package directions. A source for kelp noodles: www.rawfoodworld.com.

1 pound bean sprouts, divided
¾ cup roasted macadamia nuts, finely chopped in a
    food processor
Garnish: remaining bean sprouts, additional chopped
    macadamia nuts, sprigs of cilantro, 8 lime wedges

For the Pad Thai sauce: In a small bowl, soak the tamarind paste (remove any seeds) in the hot water for 30 minutes until soft. Place the pulp and the water in the food processor and pulse to a paste. Press the paste through a sieve into a medium saucepan. Add the salt, stevia, vinegar, and water. Boil the mixture over high heat about 10 minutes, stirring constantly. Taste for balance of flavors and remove from heat. Cool the sauce or refrigerate until ready to use.

For the salad: First shred the cabbage and place in a large bowl. Set aside.

In a wok or large frying pan, heat the sesame oil. When the oil is hot, add the dried shrimp and the chili flakes. Stir the mixture for several seconds and then add the carrots, red bell pepper, and garlic (in this order). Stir-fry the combination until the garlic is light brown.

Quickly add the cooked fish or shrimp, coconut aminos, lime juice, and the Pad Thai sauce. Mix well. Add the scallions, roasted macadamia nuts, and $1/3$ of the bean sprouts. Keep stirring until the mixture is thoroughly heated.

To serve: Place the shredded cabbage on a large platter and pour the heated salad mixture on top. Garnish with the remaining bean sprouts, macadamia nuts, cilantro sprigs, and lime wedges. Serve warm. If using the Baked Spaghetti Squash or Zucchini Noodles place on top of the cabbage before adding the warm salad mixture. Let everyone serve themselves.

Macadamia Chicken with Tangerine-Ginger Sauce

SERVES 6

Macadamia nuts, tangerines, and ginger! What an unusual and palate-pleasing combination. Serve this rich and elegant chicken dish with a light, refreshing salad and a very simply prepared green vegetable.

The Macadamia Chicken

- 3 6-ounce boned and skinned pastured or organic chicken breasts, halved
- sea salt and freshly ground pepper
- 14 ounces coconut milk, divided
- 1 cup coconut flour
- 1 cup finely ground macadamia nuts, ground in a food processor
- 2 tablespoons coconut oil
- 2 tablespoons ghee
- Garnish: sections of 3 to 4 tangerines

Tangerine-Ginger Sauce

- 1 tablespoon coconut oil
- 1 tablespoon ghee
- 1 cup yellow onion, finely minced
- 2 teaspoons minced garlic
- 2 tablespoons microplaned ginger
- ½ cup dry white wine (optional)
- ½ cup freshly squeezed tangerine juice
- remaining coconut milk
- 1 cup Chicken or Vegetable Stock (pages 102–3)

Rinse the chicken breasts with water and pat dry with paper towels. Season the breasts on both sides with salt and pepper. Set aside.

For the garnish: Peel the tangerines and remove all white pith. With a very sharp knife carefully cut in between the white dividing parts of the tangerine sections to reveal only the orange fruit. Set sections aside.

For the chicken: Preheat the oven to 375 degrees. Place 1 cup of coconut milk in a glass pie pan. Place the coconut flour in another pie pan. Place the macadamia nuts on a plate. Reserve the remaining coconut milk for the sauce.

In a large sauté pan over medium high heat, warm the coconut oil and the ghee together. Dredge the chicken breasts, first in the coconut flour, shaking off the excess, then the coconut milk. Last, press them into the macadamia nuts on both sides. Sauté the breasts on both sides until golden brown, turning carefully so you do not break the nut coating. Transfer the chicken breasts to a 9 × 13-inch glass baking dish and bake until no longer pink in the middle, about 15 minutes.

For the tangerine-ginger sauce: Wipe out the sauté pan with a paper towel and add 1 tablespoon each of the coconut oil and ghee to the pan. Over medium high heat cook the onions, garlic, and ginger, stirring often until the onions begin to brown, about 5 minutes. Add the wine, tangerine juice, and stock and reduce the liquid by half, about 8–10 minutes. Transfer the sauce to a blender and blend until smooth. Return the sauce to the pan and add the remaining coconut milk. Salt and pepper to taste.

To serve: Cut the chicken breasts in half and place on dinner plates. Also place your choice of vegetables on a plate. Spoon the sauce over the top and garnish with the tangerine sections. Serve a salad on the side.

Roast Breast of Duck
with Port Sauce & Pear Salad

8 SERVINGS

Duck is rarely served these days, but it is rich and full of flavor. Serve duck during the holidays as an alternative to turkey or ham. Serve the duck with your favorite bright green seasonal vegetable. Reserve the duck fat from the roasting pan to use as a delicious fat for cooking breakfast eggs.

The Duck

4 large duck breasts, about ¾ pound each

½ teaspoon fennel seeds

¼ teaspoon ground coriander

½ teaspoon freshly ground black pepper

2 teaspoons sea salt

zest of 1 organic orange

2 teaspoons fresh thyme leaves

¼ cup port

¼ cup freshly squeezed orange juice

The Port Sauce

1 tablespoon ghee

2 tablespoon minced shallots

½ cup chicken stock (recipe in soup section)

6 sprigs of fresh thyme leaves

zest of 2 organic oranges

1 cinnamon stick

⅛ teaspoon paprika

remaining port/orange juice mixture

pinch of sea salt and a twist of pepper

Pear Salad

2 large ripe organic pears, halved lengthwise, seeds removed, sliced ¼ inch thick

8 ounces arugula, mesclun, or watercress

½ cup toasted hazelnuts or pecans (I like hazelnuts with the duck)

½ cup fresh mint leaves, finely chopped

2 scallions, white and green parts, thinly sliced on
the diagonal

Salad Dressing

Prepare in advance.

¾ cup extra-virgin olive oil

¾ cup freshly squeezed organic orange juice

¼ cup organic pear juice

1 tablespoon Dijon mustard

½ teaspoon orange zest

¼ teaspoon sea salt and a twist of pepper

Preheat the oven to 400 degrees.

To prepare the duck breasts: Pound the fennel seeds in a morter or grind in a spice grinder and combine with the coriander, pepper, salt, orange zest, and thyme leaves. In a small bowl mix the port and orange juice. With the tip of a sharp knife, score the fat on the duck breasts in a crisscross pattern. Rub the duck breasts with a teaspoon of the port-orange juice mixture. Set the duck breasts aside on a plate. Reserve the port/orange juice mixture for the port sauce.

To cook the duck breasts: Bring a large heavy-bottomed skillet to medium-high heat. Place the duck breasts in the hot pan, skin side down, and sear until the skin is a deep golden brown and the duck fat is rendered into the pan. Turn the duck breasts over and place the skillet in the oven and continue to cook the breasts until the internal temperature reaches 135 with an instant-read thermometer, 4–8 minutes, depending on the size of the duck breasts. I like my duck medium-rare, with a little pink in the middle. When the duck breasts are done, immediately transfer to a cutting board to rest. Do not slice until the juices are settled or the duck will be dry. At this point reheat the preprepared sauce.

To make the port sauce: In a saucepan sauté the shallots in the ghee until soft. Add the stock, thyme, orange zest, cinnamon stick, paprika, and the remaining port/orange juice mixture and bring to a boil. Reduce the mixture to half of its original volume or until it reaches the consistency of a light syrup. Season with salt and pepper to taste. Remove from heat and strain the sauce. Return the sauce to the saucepan and reheat after the duck breasts are done and resting and before slicing.

For the salad dressing: In a large bowl whisk together the olive oil, orange juice, pear juice, Dijon mustard, orange zest, salt, and pepper. You will add the salad ingredients to the bowl when ready to serve the dinner.

To prep the salad: Place all the salad ingredients, except the pear slices, in a bowl and set aside until ready to add to the bowl of dressing ingredients.

To serve the dinner: While the duck is resting, and before slicing, toss the salad ingredients in the bowl with the dressing.

Divide the salad evenly onto dinner plates. Place the pear slices on top of the salad. Then, with a very sharp slicing knife, slice the duck breasts on the diagonal to get long slices. Fan the slices onto the dinner plates. Place your chosen vegetable on the plate next to the duck. Spoon the hot port sauce over the duck.

PERFECT ENDINGS

It is important today, with the increase in diabetes and our national problem of obesity, that we eliminate all potential sources of sugar from our diet. This is especially important when raising children. With the following dessert recipes we appreciate the natural, not overly sweetened, flavors of berries and other fruits. In this section I have included simple desserts that will please the sweet tooth and make a perfect ending to a wonderful meal. The recipes are gluten-free, refined sugar–free, honey-, maple syrup–, and agave-free. They are all very special and satisfyingly full of flavor.

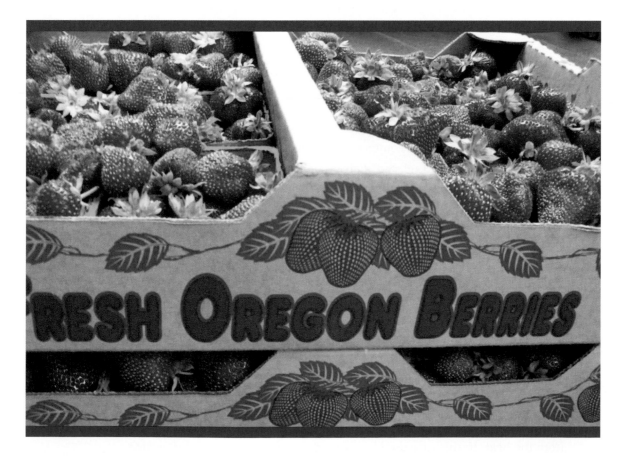

Coconut Milk Panna Cotta
with Raspberries & Raspberry Sauce

SERVES 4 TO 5

Panna cotta has a very silky texture.

The Panna Cotta

¼ cup cold water

1 packet unflavored gelatin

3½ cups coconut milk (you may also use pastured cream)

pinch of sea salt

Stevita stevia, to taste

1 teaspoon vanilla

Garnish: raspberries and sprigs of mint, optional

The Raspberry Sauce

This sauce is fresh and bright!

4 cups fresh or frozen organic raspberries

Stevita stevia, to taste

2 tablespoons fresh lemon juice

additional water, if necessary to blend

For the panna cotta: Place the cold water in a small bowl, sprinkle the gelatin over the top, and mix together. Set the gelatin mixture aside to soften.

In a medium saucepan combine the coconut milk, salt, and stevia. Over medium heat, bring to a gentle boil and then immediately remove from heat. Whisk in the gelatin and vanilla.

Divide the mixture into small dessert bowls or martini glasses. Place the glasses on a tray and cover them with plastic wrap. Refrigerate for 5–6 hours.

For the raspberry sauce: Place all the ingredients, except the water, in the food processor or blender and blend until liquefied. Add additional water in small amounts as needed. Taste for sweetness, adding more stevia if desired. Strain the mixture and refrigerate until ready to serve the dessert. It is best to use the sauce the same day you make it. Freeze leftover sauce for another time or for smoothies or your morning yogurt.

Serve the panna cotta chilled, topped with the raspberries and a drizzle of the raspberry sauce.

Variation: Omit the vanilla extract and add 2 tablespoons freshly squeezed Meyer lemon juice and 2 tablespoons grated lemon rind when you remove the coconut milk from the heat. In this case use blackberries or marionberries as the garnish.

Berry Blissful Ice Cream
MAKES ABOUT 1 QUART

*Ice cream made from coconut milk has all the richness
of real cream. I promise.*

3½ cups coconut milk
½ pound of your favorite organic strawberries,
    raspberries, marionberries, or blueberries
Stevita stevia, to taste

In a blender or food processor, puree the coconut milk, berries, and stevia until the ingredients are well blended. Refrigerate until the mixture is very cold or put it in the freezer to chill rapidly. If using frozen berries, the mixture is probably cold enough at this point.

Using an electric home ice cream machine, process the ice cream according to the manufacturer's directions. Eat immediately if not sooner.

To store the ice cream, transfer to a plastic container with a lid and place in the freezer. You may have to soften the ice cream in the refrigerator before serving it the next time.

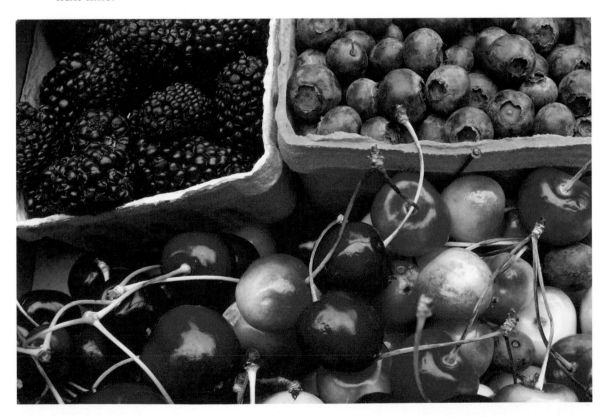

Lemon-Lime Coeur a la Crème
with Raspberry Sauce

SERVES 6

Heart of the cream is a classic dessert. It is very rich. Goat cheese gives this dessert an extra tang, like cheesecake. Normally, you would use a traditional coeur a la crème ramekin for this dessert, but I really don't think it's necessary. Do not make this dessert if you cannot have dairy.

5 ounces goat cheese

¼ cup Bellwether Farms sheep's milk ricotta (or another whole milk ricotta)

Stevita stevia, to taste

½ cup Green Valley Organics lactose-free sour sream (or another organic sour cream)

1 tablespoon each lemon and lime juice

1 teaspoon each microplaned lemon and lime zest

½ cup pastured cream

pinch of sea salt

Garnish: raspberries, Raspberry Sauce (page 244) and sprigs of mint

In a food processor combine the goat cheese, ricotta, stevia, sour cream, lemon and lime juices, and zests. Blend until smooth, scraping the mixture from the sides of the bowl as needed. Remove to a large bowl.

In a separate bowl whip the cream and a pinch of salt with a whisk or electric beater until stiff peaks form. Add the whipped cream to the goat cheese mixture in three separate additions, folding well each time, until the whipped cream is completely incorporated.

Divide the mixture by spoonfuls into martini glasses or pretty goblets. Serve immediately garnished with the raspberries, a drizzle of sauce, and a sprig of mint. You can make the Coeur a la Crème in advance and refrigerate until ready to serve.

Variation: Omit the lemon and lime juices and zests and add a teaspoon of vanilla or your favorite liqueur. Sliced ripe nectarines or peaches would also be beautiful as a garnish.

Nora's Coconut Bliss Truffles

MAKES A LOT!

I adapted Nora Gedgaudas's recipe for these delicious, trufflelike morsels. Because I've always craved cookies and candy, these are the perfect solution to the problem of what to eat instead. I've tried them out on all my friends and they agree: they are richly satisfying and fill the bill when the sweet tooth needs soothing. Now I eat these instead of a cookie when I get cravings for sweets. Just to let you know, the truffles must be stored in the refrigerator. Toasting the nuts and coconut makes a huge difference in the flavor.

2 cups almonds, pecans, or pistachios, toasted

8 ounces pastured butter, ghee, or coconut oil

2 cups organic almond butter or another nut butter
   (no peanut butter, it is a legume)

1 cup organic coconut flour (or for chocolate truffles,
   substitute ½ cup coconut flour and ½ cup organic
   cocoa powder*)

1 cup organic dried coconut, lightly toasted

1 cup your choice of ground seeds (flax, sesame, or chia)

1 tablespoon vanilla

½ teaspoon sea salt or to taste

Preheat the oven to 400 degrees. Place the nuts on a sheet pan and toast in the oven, stirring occasionally, to evenly toast the nuts.

After toasting, grind the nuts very finely in a food processor. Also in a food processor blend together the butter and almond butter. Blend in the coconut flour. Transfer the mixture to a large bowl and mix in the remaining ingredients, blending thoroughly. With a spoon, portion the mixture into balls the size of a small walnut. They don't have to be completely round, because truffles are misshapen anyway. For added flair, roll the truffles in organic unsweetened cocoa powder, toasted coconut, or finely ground nuts (try finely ground macadamia nuts). Store the truffles in an airtight container in the refrigerator.

This recipe will make a lot of truffles. You can serve them at your next party (in small paper candy cups) Eat the truffles when the mood strikes you. The mood strikes me about three times a day and I don't leave the house without a truffle. They definitely cut the cravings for sweets.

---

*Try raw organic cocoa powder. There are sources online.

Lemon Cheesecake with Berries

SERVES 8

This lovely, lemon-scented cheesecake is made with goat's milk chevre and sheep's milk ricotta. The slightly tart flavor of the chevre makes this cheesecake very special. Serve with your favorite ripe summer berries. In the winter you can warm frozen berries and spoon them over the top of the cheesecake when you serve it.

The Crust

2½ cups pecans

3 tablespoons ghee or coconut oil

⅛ teaspoon sea salt

¼ teaspoon vanilla

1 tablespoon warm water if needed

The Filling

5 ounces Meyenberg Crème de Chevre* (or cream cheese)

8 ounces Bellwether Farms sheep's milk ricotta (or another whole milk ricotta)

½ cup Capretta Rich and Creamy Goat Yogurt

2 eggs

Stevita stevia, to taste

1 teaspoon lemon zest

juice of 1 lemon

pinch of sea salt

Garnish: blackberries, raspberries, strawberries, or blueberries; sprigs of mint

Preheat the oven to 400 degrees.

For the crust: In a food processor grind the pecans until fine, add the ghee, salt, and vanilla and a tablespoon of water. Pulse until the mixture holds together and is moist. Add a little more water, if necessary. Pat the nut crust into a 9-inch glass pie pan and lightly toast in the oven 5–10 minutes, checking frequently. Do not let the crust get too dark.

---

*Meyenberg Crème de Chevre is a goat cream cheese. Because it may not be readily available everywhere, as a substitute use regular goat cheese thinned slightly with cream, or just use organic cream cheese. I like the flavor of the goat cheese, however.

For the filling: Rinse out the food processor and add the crème de chevre, ricotta, yogurt, eggs, stevia, lemon zest, lemon juice, and salt. Blend the mixture until smooth, scraping the the sides of the bowl as needed. Pour the cheesecake filling into the toasted crust.

Reduce the oven temperature to 325 degrees. Place the cheesecake in a 9 × 13-inch baking dish, half-filled with hot water. Place the cheesecake and baking dish in the oven. Bake the cheesecake for approximately 40 minutes, or until just set. Remove from the oven and refrigerate for about 5–6 hours.

To serve: Slice the cheesecake and place on pretty dessert plates. Garnish with the berries and a sprig of mint.

Pears Stuffed with Chevre

SERVES 2

So simple! This makes a wonderful holiday dessert. The goat's milk chevre is deliciously tangy. If you want a milder flavor, use sheep's milk ricotta instead of chevre or just use organic cream cheese.

2 ripe pears (Bartlett) or another favorite seasonal
   pear
2 tablespoons late-harvest white wine
6 tablespoons Meyenberg Crème de Chevre or
   Bellwether Farms sheep's milk ricotta
juice of ½ lemon, preferably a Meyer lemon
¼ teaspoon grated lemon zest
Garnish: organic cocoa powder or grated 85%
   organic chocolate bar, pomegranate seeds

Peel the pears and cut them in half lengthwise. Remove the cores with a spoon. Rub the surface of the halves with lemon to prevent discoloration.

In a bowl whisk together the wine, chevre, lemon juice, and zest. Spoon the cheese mixture into the hollow part of the pear halves. Place the two halves on two dessert plates and dust with cocoa powder or grated chocolate. Pomegranate seeds sprinkled around the plate are very festive.

I Am Bright Avocado-Lime Pie

MAKES ONE 9-INCH PIE

This refreshingly tart pie is a beautiful light green color and will certainly impress guests. The crust adds a wonderful, nutty complement to the silky texture of the filling.

The Coconut-Pecan Crust*

1¼ cups pecans

¼ teaspoon vanilla

⅛ teaspoon sea salt

3 tablespoons coconut oil or ghee

1 tablespoon warm water, if needed

1¼ cups unsweetened organic shredded coconut

The Avocado-Lime Filling

¾ cup lime juice

zest of 1 lime

Stevita stevia, to taste

1 cup mashed avocado (ripe, but no dark spots)

¼ cup coconut milk, or more, if necessary

2 teaspoons vanilla

⅛ teaspoon sea salt

¾ cup coconut oil, melted

Garnish: 1 lime, thinly sliced; sprigs of mint

Preheat the oven to 375 degrees.

For the crust: In the bowl of a food processor pulse the pecans, vanilla, and salt until fine. Continue processing while adding the coconut oil or ghee and warm water until the crust mixture sticks together. Remove the mixture to a bowl and add the shredded coconut. Mix well and press crust into a greased 9-inch glass pie pan. Place the pie crust in the oven and toast, 5–10 minutes, watching carefully so crust does not burn.

For the avocado-lime filling: In the food processor, blend all ingredients, except the warm coconut oil, until smooth. With the processor running, slowly add the

---

*For your breakfast bar tray you can make the recipe of nut crust and toast it in the oven on a sheet pan until light brown. Use the mixture to sprinkle on breakfast yogurt, fruit, or other desserts.

warm coconut oil, blending until well incorporated. The mixture will emulsify like mayonnaise. Pour the filling into the prepared crust and refrigerate until firm.

   To serve: Slice the pie and place on pretty dessert plates. Garnish with the slices of lime and the mint sprigs.

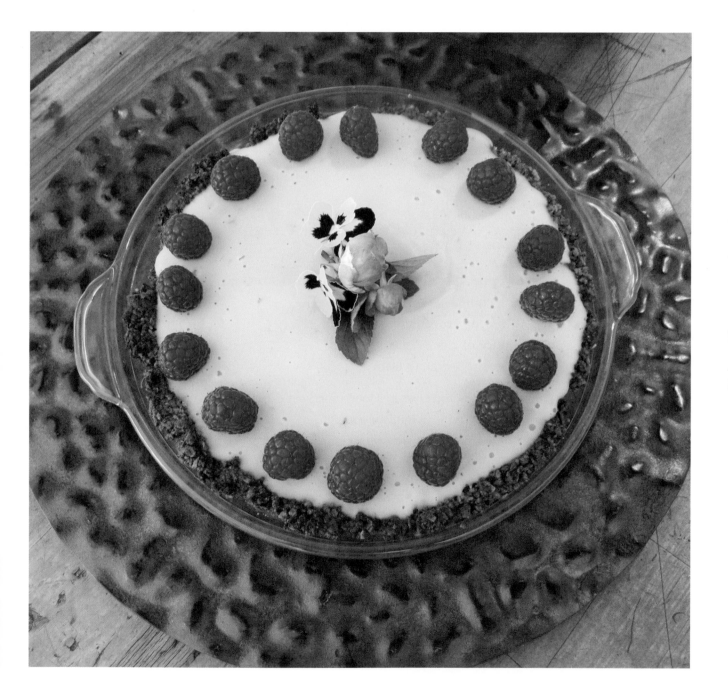

Peaches and Cream Ice Cream

MAKES ABOUT 1 QUART

3½ cups pastured cream or coconut milk, chilled

½ pound chilled ripe summer peaches or nectarines,
   skins removed and diced

Stevita stevia, to taste

1 teaspoon vanilla extract

In a blender or food processor, puree the cream or coconut milk, peaches, stevia, and vanilla until well blended.

Using your home electric ice cream machine, process the ice cream according to the manufacturer's directions. Serve immediately.

Avocado-Coconut Ice Cream

MAKES ABOUT 1 QUART

3 ripe (no brown spots) medium-size avocados,
   chilled

3½ cups coconut milk, chilled

juice of 2 or 3 limes

Stevita stevia, to taste

Peel and pit the avocados and place in a food processor. Add the chilled coconut milk, lime juice, and stevia and blend until smooth.

Using your home electric ice cream machine, process the ice cream according to the manufacturer's directions. Serve immediately.

San Joaquin Cantaloupe Ice

SERVES 6

I grew up in the Cantaloupe Capitol of the World: Coalinga, California. When the melons were too ripe to ship, we could buy a crate of sweet, vine-ripened cantaloupe for one dollar. For this recipe, find the sweetest late-summer melon you can. Coalinga, by the way, is also the Horned Toad Capitol of the World.

> 3 pounds ripe, sweet cantaloupe or another favorite
>   late-harvest melon
> 2 tablespoons lime juice, or 2 tablespoons late-
>   harvest white wine
> 1 teaspoon microplaned lime zest
> Garnish: 2 tablespoons unsalted pistachios, toasted
>   and chopped

Remove the rind from the melon, halve the melon, and remove the seeds. Cut the melon into chunks and puree the flesh in a food processor until liquefied. Add the lime juice and zest and blend briefly to incorporate. Freeze the mixture in an ice cream maker according to the manufacturer's directions. Serve immediately.

To serve, divide the cantaloupe ice into widemouth wine goblets. Sprinkle chopped pistachios on top of the dessert.

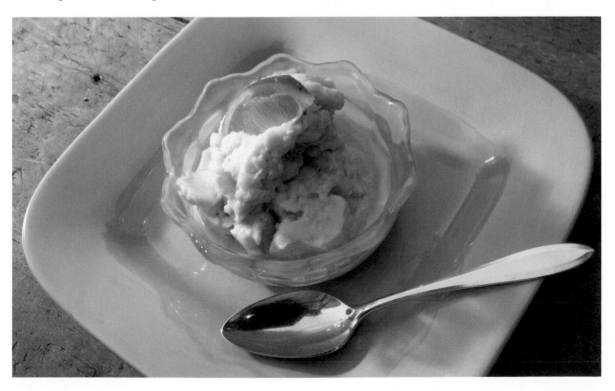

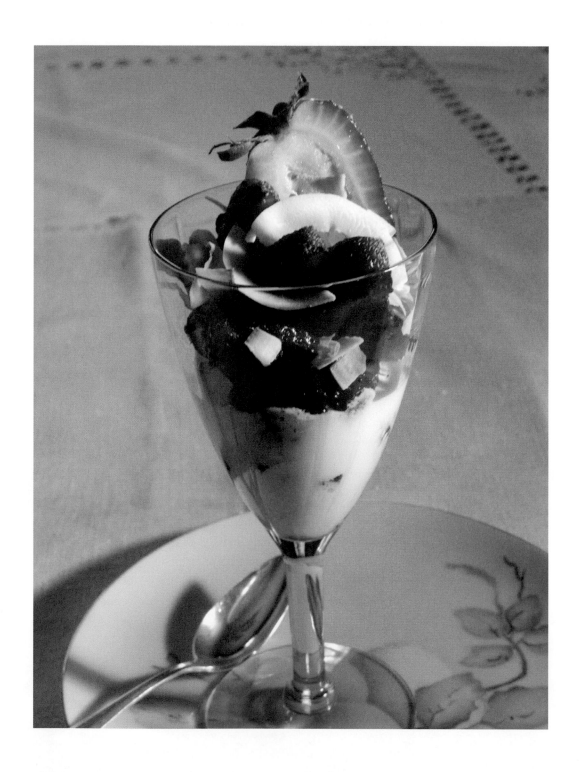

Berries with Toasted Coconut Sauce

SERVES 4

Summer is berry time and this is a very luxurious way to serve them.
This very simple recipe would make a special brunch dessert.

The Coconut Sauce

½ cup plus 4 tablespoons shredded or flaked organic
    coconut (unsweetened)

2 cups coconut milk

Stevita stevia, to taste

1 teaspoon vanilla

The Berries

4 cups organic strawberries, sliced (marionberries,
    raspberries, or peaches will work)

Garnish: 4 tablespoons toasted coconut, sprigs of mint

Preheat the oven to 375 degrees.

For the sauce: Place the coconut on a sheet pan and toast in the oven until light brown, about 5 minutes. Stir often to toast evenly. Remove coconut from oven and reserve 4 tablespoons for the garnish.

In a bowl whisk together the coconut milk, stevia, and vanilla until well blended. Stir in a half cup of the toasted coconut. You can chill the sauce or serve it at room temperature.

To serve: Spoon some of the sauce on the bottom of each of 4 dessert bowls or widemouth wineglasses and then divide the berries on top of the sauce. Spoon some more sauce over the berries. Sprinkle the remaining toasted coconut on top of each dessert. Beautiful!

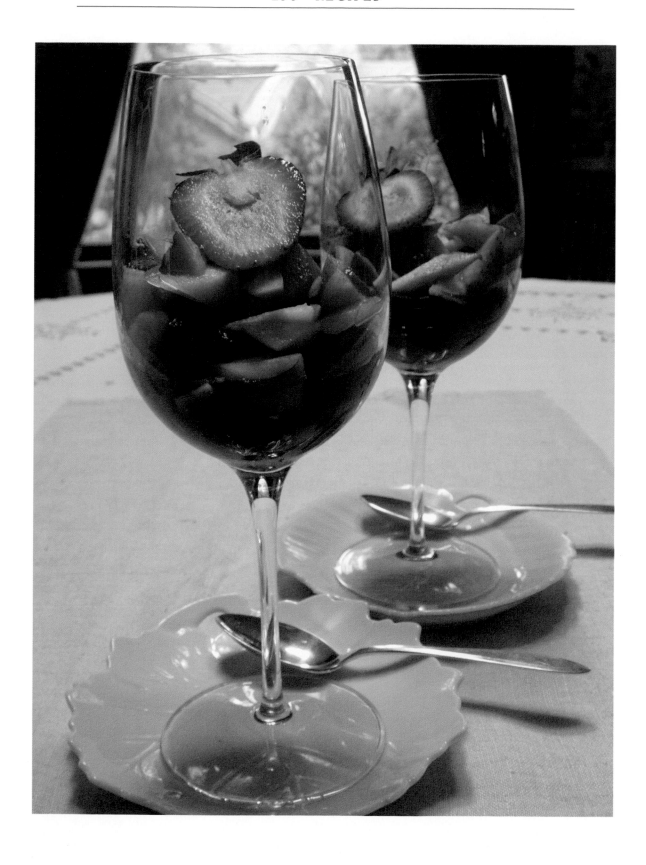

Strawberries and Nectarines with Balsamic Vinegar

SERVES 6

This combination of fruit and lightly sprinkled balsamic vinegar is a sensational way to end a meal.

The Sauce

    2 tablespoons aged balsamic vinegar*

    2 tablespoons water

    1 cup organic strawberries

The Fruit

    3 cups organic strawberries, sliced

    3 cups organic nectarines, sliced

    twist of black pepper, optional

For the sauce: In a small saucepan bring to a boil the water, balsamic vinegar, and the strawberries. Cook, while stirring, for 1–2 minutes. Remove from heat and let sit.

For the fruit: In a large bowl combine the sliced strawberries and nectarines. Toss the fruit in the hot strawberry-balsamic syrup and the optional black pepper. Let the fruit stand, stirring occasionally, until ready to serve.

Serve the dessert in martini glasses or widemouth wineglasses.

---

*The selection of specially flavored aged balsamic vinegars at Olive Oil and Beyond is fantastic: www .oliveoilandbeyond.com.

RESOURCES

Spices

Celtic Sea Salt: www.celticseasalt.com

Frontier Natural Products Co-Op:
   www.frontiernaturalbrands.com

Organic Planet: www.organic-planet.com

Organic Oils

Aunt Patty's Organic Extra Virgin
   Coconut Oil: www.AuntPattys.com

Bariani Organic Olive Oil:
   www.barianioliveoil.com

Barlean's Organic Oils:
   www.barleans.com

California Estate Olive Oil and Market:
   www.caloliveoil.com

Gold Label Virgin Coconut Oil
   from the Philippines:
   www.tropicaltraditions.com

Inesscents, 100% African Shea Butter
   and (scented oils): www.inesscents.com

J Le Blanc Nut Oils from Burgundy,
   France: www.klkellerimports.com

Long Meadow Ranch: Napa Valley,
   Organic Olive Oils:
   www.longmeadowranch.com

McEvoy Ranch Olive Oils:
   www.mcevoyranch.com

Organic Sesame Oil:
   www.edenfoods.com

Ultimate Superfoods, 100% organic
   Real Raw Cacao Butter:
   www.UltimateSuperfoods.com

Organic Nuts

Braga Organic Farms Bulk Organic Nuts:
   www.buyorganicnuts.com

D&S Ranches:
   www.california-almonds.com

Freddy Guys Oregon Hazelnuts:
   www.freddyguys.com

McAfee Farms, Organic Pastures,
   Truly Raw almonds:
   www.organicpastures.com

Chocolate

Raw Organic Cocoa Powder, Sunfood:
   www.sunfood.com

Tropical Traditions:
   www.tropicaltraditions.com

Z Natural, Raw Organic Cacao Powder:
   www.ZNaturalFoods.com

**Environmentally Responsible
Seafood Sources and Information**

Blue Ocean Institute: www.blueocean.org

Ecofish: www.ecofish.com

Environmental Defense Fund: www.edf.org

Monterey Bay Aquarium: www.monterey
   bayaquarium.or/cr/seafoodwatch.aspx

Grassfed and Pasture-Raised Meats

Beelers Pure Pork:
  www.beelerspurepork.com
Community Supported Agriculture
  (CSA): www.csacenter.org
Eat Well Guide: www.eatwellguide.org
Eat Wild: www.eatwild.com (look for the
  producers in your state)
Grassfed Association:
  www.american grassfed.or/producers.htm
Heritage Foods USA:
  www.heritagefoodsusa.com
Llano Seco Organic Pork:
  www.llanoseco.com
Nevada County Free-Range Beef:
  www.nevadacountyfreerangebeef.com
U.S. Wellness Meats:
  www.grasslandbeef.com

Game Meats

Buffalo: www.organicbuffalo.com;
  www.eatwild.com;
  www.buffalogroves.com
Duck, turkey game birds, pheasant,
  rabbit: www.dartagnan.com
Venison, antelope, wild boar:
  www.brokenarrowranch.com
Yak: www.yakmeat.us

Eggs, Poultry, and Dairy

Ancient Organics:
  www.ancientorganics.com
The California Artisan Cheese Guild:
  www.cacheeseguild.org
Green Valley Organics, lactose-free:
  www.greenvalleylactosefree.com
Hoffman Hatchery, Inc.:
  www.hoffmanhatchery.com

Liberty Ducks, Sonoma County, Calif.:
  www.libertyducks.com
Marin Sun Farms:
  www.cuesa.org/farm/marin-sun.farms
Meyenberg Dairy goat's milk products:
  www.meyenberg.com
Organic Pastures Raw Dairy:
  www.organicpastures.com
Pure Indian Foods, 100% pasture fed
  ghee: www.pureindianfoods.com
Willie Bird Turkeys, Sonoma, County
  Calif.: www.williebird.com

Other Organic Websites

Livin Spoonful, sprouted crackers:
  www.livingspoonful.com
Lydia's Organics, sprouted seed crackers:
  www.lydiasorganics.com
Organic Moringa:
  www.organicmoringausa.com
Radiant Life:
  www.radiantlifecatalog.com
Wilderness Family Naturals:
  www.wildernessfamilynaturals.com

Garden Seeds

Baker Creek: www.rareseeds.com
Native American Seed:
  www.seedsource.com
Native Seed Network:
  www.nativeseednetwork.org
Seeds of Change:
  www.seedsofchange.com
Seed Savers Exchange: www.seedsavers.org

Pure Water

Berkey Water Filteration Systems:
  www.berkeyfilters.com

Organizations for Further Research

Celiac.com: www.celiac.com

Campaign for Real Milk:
   www.realmilk.com

Dr. Mercola website: www.Mercola.com

Fair Trade Resource Network:
   www.fairtraderesource.org

Food Democracy Now:
   www.fooddemocracynow.org

Food Routes: www.foodroutes.org

The Future of Food DVD by Lily Films:
   www.futureoffood.com

Genetically Engineered Food Alert:
   www.gefoodalert.org or call
   800-390-3373

HeartGate Sanctuary: www.inei-re.org

Institute for Responsible Technology:
   www.instituteforresponsibletechnology.org

Organization for World Food Supply
   Issues: www.foodfirst.com

Orthomolecular Health:
   www.orthomolecularhealth.com

The Pfeiffer Treatment Center,
   *Nutritional Treatment for Mental
   Disorders*: www.hriptc.com

Polyface Farms: www.polyfacefarms.com

Price Pottenger Nutritional Foundation:
   www.ppnf.org

School of Creation:
   www.schoolofcreation.com

Seed Magazine, *The Journal of Organic
   Living*

The Soil Association:
   www.soilassociation.com

Weston A. Price Foundation:
   www.WestonAPrice.org

Union of Concerned Scientists:
   www.uscusa.org

American Raw Milk Cheese

Organic Pastures Raw Dairy, California:
   Truly Raw Cheddar

Pt. Reyes Farmstead Cheese Company,
   California: Cow's milk, Raw Holstein
   Original Blue, Blue Cheese Crumbles

Organic Valley Dairy, Wisconsin: Cow's
   milk, raw milk and cream, original raw
   butter (pastured)

Green Pastures Dairy, Minnesota: Cow's
   milk cheese, Minnesota Farmstead
   Raw Gouda

Rumiano, California: Cow's milk
   cheeses, raw cheddar, raw monterey
   jack, raw Swiss

Mt. Sterling, Wisconsin: goat cheeses,
   raw milk cheddar, raw milk sharp
   cheddar, raw milk smoked cheddar, a
   variety of flavored raw goat jack cheese,
   raw goat milk feta, raw goat mozzarella

Redwood Hill Farm, California: Goat's
   milk cheese, Sonoma County raw goat
   feta

Sierra Nevada Cheese Company,
   California: Goat's milk cheeses, raw
   goat milk monterey Jacques, capre raw
   aged goat cheddar

Imported Raw Milk Cheeses

Whole Foods: Buenalba with wine, raw
   goat cheese, Papillon Roquefort, raw
   sheep's cheese

Trader Joe's: Swiss raw milk gruyere

RECOMMENDED BOOKS AND PUBLICATIONS

Allport, Susan. *The Queen of Fats: Why Omega-3s Were Removed from the Western Diet and What We Can Do to Replace Them.* Berkeley: University of California Press, 2006.

Boyd Eaton, S., Marjorie Shostak, and Melvin Konner. *The Paleolithic Prescription.* New York: Harper and Row, 1988.

Brandysiewicz, Ania. *Consiousness and the Enlightened Body.* Santa Clara, Calif.: DeHart's Media Service, 2010.

Braly, James, and Ron Hoggan. *Dangerous Grains.* New York: Viking, 2002.

Campbell-McBride, Natasha. *Gut and Psychology Syndrome: Natural Treatment for Autism, Dyspraxia, ADD/HD, Dylexia, Depression, and Schizophrenia.* Middle River, Md: International Nutrition, 1988.

Cohen, Mark Nathan. *The Food Crisis in Prehistory: Overpopulation and the Origins of Agriculture.* New Haven, Conn.: Yale University Press, 1977.

Davis, William. *Wheat Belly.* New York: Rodale Books, 2011.

Diamond, Jared. *Collapse.* New York: Viking, 2005.

———. *Guns, Germs and Steel.* New York: Norton, 2005.

Fallon, Sally. *Nourishing Traditions: The Cookbook That Challenges Politically Correct Nutrition and the Diet Dictocrats.* Washington, D.C.: NewTrends, 1999.

Fallon, Sally, and Mary Enig. *Eat Fat, Lose Fat.* New York: Hudson Street Press, 2005.

Gedgaudas, Nora T. *Primal Body, Primal Mind: Beyond the Paleo Diet for Total Health and a Longer Life.* Rochester, Vt.: Healing Arts Press, 2011.

Hemenway, Toby. *Gaia's Garden: A Guide to Home-Scale Permaculture.* White River Junction, Vt., Chelsea Green, 2009.

Hoffer, Abram. *Orthomolecular Medicine for Everyone.* Laguna Beach, CA: 2008.

———. *Smart Nutrients: Prevent and Treat Alzheimer's, Enhance Brain Function.* Ridgefield, Conn.: Vital Health, 2002.

Hyman, Mark. *The UltraMind Solution.* New York: Scribner, 2008.

Keith, Lierre. *The Vegetarian Myth: Food, Justice and Sustainability.* Crescent City, Calif.: Flashpoint, 2009.

Kilarski, Barbara. *Keep Chickens! Tending Small Flocks in Cities, Suburbs, and Other Small Spaces.* North Adams, Mass.: Storey, 2003.

Kingsolver, Barbara. *Animal Vegetable, Miracle.* New York: HarperCollins, 2007.

Lipton, Bruce H. *The Biology of Belief: Unleashing the Power of Consciousness, Matter and Miracles.* Carlsbad, Calif.: Hay House, 2008.

Merkel, Jim. *Radical Simplicity: Small Footprints on a Finite Earth.* Gabriola Island, B.C.: New Society Publishers, 2003.

Pheiffer, Carl C. *Nutrition and Mental Illness.* Rochester, Vt.: Healing Arts Press, 1987.

Pollan, Michael. *In Defense of Food.* New York: Penguin, 2008.

———. *The Omnivore's Dilemma.* New York: Penguin, 2006.

Pottenger Jr., Francis Marion. *Pottenger's Cats: A Study in Nutrition.* La Mesa, Calif.: Price-Pottenger Nutrition Foundation, 2005.

Price, Weston A. *Nutrition and Physical Degeneration.* New York: Paul Hoeber, 1939.

Salatin, Joel. *Everything I Want to Do Is Illegal.* Swoope, Va.: Polyface, 2007.

———. *You Can Farm: The Entrepreneur's Guide to Start and Succeed in a Farm Enterprise.* Swoope, Va.: Polyface, 1998.

———. *The Sheer Ecstasy of Being a Lunatic Farmer.* Swoope, Va.: Polyface, 2010.

Shaw, William. *Biological Treatments for Autism and PDD.* Great Plains, Kans.: Great Plains Laboratory, Inc., 2002.

Schwarzbein, Diana. *The Schwarzbein Principle.* Deerfield Beach, Fla.: Health Communications, 2004.

Shanahan, Cate, and Luke Shanahan. *Deep Nutrition: Why Your Genes Need Traditional Food.* Lawai, Hawaii: Big Box Book, 2009.

Smith, Jeffrey. *Seeds of Deception: Exposing Industry and Government Lies about the Safety of the Genetically Engineered Foods You're Eating.* White River Junction, Vt.: 2003.

Weinstein, Jay. *The Ethical Gourmet.* New York: Broadway Books, 2006.

Wilshire, Howard G., Jane E. Nielson, and Richard W. Hazlett. *The American West at Risk: Science, Myths, and Politics of Land Abuse and Recovery.* New York: Oxford University Press, 2008.

Woodford, Keith. *Devil in the Milk: Illness, Health, and the Politics of A1 and A2 Milk.* White River Junction, Vt.: Chelsea Green, 2007.

INDEX

Rich and Spicy Italian Tomato
Sauce, 154
Roast Breast of Duck with Port
Sauce & Pear Salad, 240–42
Roasted Garlic, 85
Roasted Garlic Vinaigrette, 124
Roasted Vegetable Napoleons
with Basil Pesto, 158–59
Roasted Winter Vegetables, 172
romano cheese, 74, 77, 160–61

salad dressings
about, 119
Blue Cheese Dressing, 120
bottled, 43
Caesar Dressing, 134
Chipotle Chili Dressing,
144–45
Chipotle-Lime Dressing, 150
Citrus Vinaigrette, 121
Ginger Dressing, 132–33
Green Goddess Dressing,
140–41
Lemon Dressing, 147
Lemon Oregano Dressing, 121
Lime Dressing, 200
mayonnaise for, 123
Poppyseed Dressing, 122
Ranch Dressing, 122
Roasted Garlic Vinaigrette, 124
Spicy Ginger Dressing, 148–49
Salad of Grilled Vegetables with
Feta Cheese, 126–27
salads, 119–50
Barbecued Chicken Salad,
128–29
Beef Carpaccio Salad, 138–39
Breast of Duck with Port Sauce
& Pear Salad, 240–42
Broccoli Rabe and Feta Salad,
125
Caesar Salad, 134–35
Chicken Sausage Salad, 143
Colorful Cobb Salad, 137
Crab and Grapefruit Salad with
Microgreens & Herbs, 131

Green Goddess Salad, 140–41
Grilled Mexican Steak
Salad with Chipotle Chili
Dressing, 144–45
Heirloom Tomato Caprese
Salad, 141
Japanese Salad, 139
Mediterranean Spinach & Feta
Salad with Lemon Dressing,
147
Mexican Cole Slaw with
Chipotle-Lime Dressing, 150
Pastured Egg Salad, 129
Sautéed Chicken Livers with
Summer Greens, 132–33
Savory Green Salad, 124
Seafood Salad with Mangoes,
Avocado & Meyer Lemon
Vinaigrette, 132–33
Thai Salad with Spicy Ginger
Dressing, 148–49
Turkey Salad with Apple &
Mint, 130
salmon
Salmon Niçoise with Haricots
Verts & Pastured Eggs,
186–87
Salmon Rillettes, 96
Salmon with Avocado Slices &
Lime Dressing, 200
Salmon with Pistachio Sauce
& Grilled Vegetables, 188
Salmon with Yogurt-Dill
Sauce, 181
Smoked Salmon with Spicy
Mango Salsa, 95
Salmon with Avocado Slices &
Lime Dressing, 200
Salmon Niçoise with Haricots
Verts & Pastured Eggs,
186–87
Salmon with Pistachio Sauce &
Grilled Vegetables, 188
Salmon Rillettes, 96
Salmon with Yogurt-Dill Sauce,
181

salsas
Chili Rellenos with Fresh
Herb Salsa, 174–75
Cilantro Chicken with
Tomato-Avocado Salsa,
234–35
Flank Steak with Salsa Verde,
202–3
Pacific Rim Tuna Salsa, 92
Salsa Verde, 202–3
Scallop Ceviche with Avocado-
Mango Salsa & Belgian
Endive, 100
Smoked Salmon with Spicy
Mango Salsa, 95
Salsa Verde, 202–3
salt, 41, 50–51
San Joaquin Cantaloupe Ice, 253
Sante Fe Chipotle Chili Soup
with Lime Cream, 108–9
Sartell, Charles, 6
saturated fat, 12–15
sauces, 151–56
Asian Dipping Sauce, 227
Creole Remoulade Sauce,
194–95
Garlic Aioli, 152
Hollandaise Sauce, 71
Lemon-Caper Sauce, 232–33
Lime Dipping Sauce, 183
Pecorino Hollandaise Sauce,
77
Pistachio Sauce, 188–89
Port Sauce, 240–42
Raspberry Sauce, 246
Rich and Spicy Italian Tomato
Sauce, 154
Tangerine-Ginger Sauce,
238–39
Very Green Herb Sauce, 156
Yogurt-Dill Sauce, 181
sausages, 43–44, 143
Sautéed Broccoli Rabe with
Pecorino Romano, 160–61
Sautéed Chicken Livers with
Summer Greens, 133